Advanced Comparative Vertebrate Anatomy

Advanced Comparative Vertebrate Anatomy

Dr. P.K. Taneja

Oxford Book Company
Jaipur ▪ New Delhi

Published By

Oxford Book Company

Regd. Off. "Bony Residency", Gate No. 2
Opp. Tilak Public School, Vishweswariya Nagar,
Gopalpura Road, Jaipur - 302018, India
Ph: 0141 - 2761280, Telefax: 2761381
email - oxfordbookjpr@gmail.com
website - oxfordbookcompany.com

Delhi Office: 102, 1st Floor, Satyam House,
4327/3, Ansari Road, Darya Ganj,
New Delhi - 110002, India
Ph: 011-45652440

Distributed By

KEYA INTERNATIONAL PRESS LLP

E-mail: keyainternationalpressllp@gmail.com

First published in India, 2025

ISBN : 978-93-5524-188-7

Typeset by Shivangi Computers, Jaipur

Printed and bound in India by Thomson Press Ltd.,
New Delhi

Contents

Preface

The field of vertebrate anatomy is an ever-evolving domain that bridges the gap between classical morphological studies and modern evolutionary biology. Advanced Comparative Vertebrate Anatomy is designed to provide a comprehensive and detailed analysis of vertebrate structures, emphasizing both their functional significance and evolutionary transformations. This book aims to be an essential resource for students, researchers, and educators seeking to understand the complex interplay between form, function, and phylogeny in vertebrates.

Comparative anatomy is fundamental to the study of biological sciences, revealing the evolutionary relationships among various vertebrate groups. This book delves into the structural adaptations that define vertebrate classes, from primitive jawless fish to highly specialized mammals. It systematically explores the similarities and differences across taxa, focusing on skeletal, muscular, nervous, circulatory, respiratory, and reproductive systems. By integrating classical anatomical studies with contemporary research, this work presents an enriched perspective on the mechanisms that have shaped vertebrate evolution over millions of years.

A distinguishing feature of this book is its emphasis on functional morphology and adaptive significance. Each chapter meticulously examines how structural modifications have allowed vertebrates to thrive in diverse ecological niches. From the aerodynamic adaptations of birds to the aquatic specializations of marine mammals, the book elucidates how anatomical transformations have driven evolutionary success. Furthermore, modern advances in imaging techniques, molecular biology, and paleontological discoveries are incorporated to provide a holistic understanding of vertebrate anatomy.

The organization of the book ensures a logical progression of topics, facilitating a deeper grasp of anatomical complexities. Richly illustrated diagrams and comparative tables enhance comprehension, making intricate concepts accessible to a broad readership. This book aspires to serve as a definitive guide, fostering curiosity and inspiring further exploration in the fascinating world of vertebrate anatomy.

— ***Dr. P.K. Taneja***

Chapter 1

Mammal Vertebrates

***Mammals (Class Mammalia (Pron:** /mYÈmejli.Y/))* are a clade of warm-blooded amniotes. Among the features that distinguish them from the other amniotes, the reptiles and the birds, are hair, three middle ear bones, mammary glands in females, and a neocortex (a region of the brain). The mammalian brain regulates body temperature and the circulatory system, including the four-chambered heart.

The mammals include the largest animals on the planet, the rorqual whales, as well as the most intelligent, the apes. The basic body type is a four-legged land-borne animal, but some mammals are adapted for life at sea, in the air, in the trees, or on two legs. The largest group of mammals, the placentals, have a placenta which feeds the offspring during pregnancy. Mammals range in size from the 30–40 millimetre (1- to 1.5-inch) bumblebee bat to the 33-metre (108-foot) blue whale.

The word "mammal" is modern, from the scientific name *Mammalia* coined by Carl Linnaeus in 1758, derived from the Latin *mamma* ("teat, pap"). All female mammals nurse their young with milk, which is secreted from special glands, the mammary glands. According to *Mammal Species of the World*, 5,702 species were known in 2005. These were grouped in 1,229 genera, 153 families and 29 orders. In 2008 the IUCN completed a five-year, 17,000-scientist Global Mammal Assessment for its IUCN Red List, which counted 5,488 accepted species at the end of that period. In some classifications, the mammals are divided into two subclasses (not counting fossils): the Prototheria (order of Monotremata) and the Theria, the latter composed of the infraclasses Metatheria and Eutheria. The marsupials comprise the crown group of the Metatheria and therefore include all living metatherians as well as many extinct ones; the placentals likewise constitute the crown group of the Eutheria.

Except for the five species of monotremes (which lay eggs), all living mammals give birth to live young. Most mammals, including the six most species-rich orders, belong to the placental group. The three largest orders, in descending order, are Rodentia (mice, rats, porcupines, beavers, capybaras, and other gnawing mammals), Chiroptera (bats), and Soricomorpha (shrews, moles and solenodons).

The next three largest orders, depending on the classification scheme used, are the primates, to which the human species belongs, the Cetartiodactyla (including the even-toed hoofed mammals and the whales), and the Carnivora (cats, dogs, weasels, bears, seals, and their relatives). While the classification of mammals at the family level has been relatively stable, different treatments at higher levels—subclass, infraclass, and order—appear in contemporaneous literature, especially for the marsupials. Much recent change has reflected the results of cladistic analysis and molecular genetics. Results from molecular genetics, for example, have led to the adoption of new groups such as the Afrotheria and the abandonment of traditional groups such as the Insectivora. The early synapsid mammalian ancestors were sphenacodont pelycosaurs, a group that also included *Dimetrodon*. At the end of the Carboniferous period, this group diverged from the sauropsid line that led to today's reptiles and birds. Preceded by many diverse groups of non-mammalian synapsids (sometimes referred to as mammal-like reptiles), the first mammals appeared in the early Mesozoic era. The modern mammalian orders arose in the Paleogene and Neogene periods of the Cenozoic era.

Varying Definitions, Varying Dates

In an influential 1988 paper, Timothy Rowe defined Mammalia phylogenetically as the crown group mammals, the clade consisting of the most recent common ancestor of living monotremes (echidnas and platypuses) and therian mammals (marsupials and placentals) and all descendants of that ancestor. A broader phylogenetic definition was provided in a 2004 book by Kielan-Jaworowska, Cifelli, and Luo, who defined Mammalia as the clade originating with the most recent common ancestor, not only of the monotremes and the therians, but also of *Sinoconodon*, the morganucodonts, and the docodonts.

The morganucodonts and the docodonts, included by Rowe in the unranked clade Mammaliaformes, had a widespread distribution in the northern continents and had many of the characteristics that traditionally would have classified them as mammals. In particular, some docodonts were furry. Finally, many paleontologists define Mammalia based on skeletal characteristics rather than ancestral relations; *Adelobasileus* is included on this basis, though this animal satisfies neither Rowe's definition nor that of Kielan-Jaworowska *et al.*

Mammalia, considered as the crown group, appeared in the Pliensbachian age of the early Jurassic period. In the broader sense given to the term by Kielan-Jaworowska *et al.*, the group arose in the Carnian age at the beginning of the Late Triassic. Mammalia is no older if defined by skeletal characteristics; *Adelobasileus*, the earliest animal that is included on this basis, is also dated to the Carnian. In any case, the temporal range of the group extends to the present day.

Distinguishing Features

Living mammal species can be identified by the presence of sweat glands, including those that are specialised to produce milk to nourish their young.

In classifying fossils, however, other features must be used, since soft tissue glands and many other features are not visible in fossils..

Many traits shared by all living mammals appeared among the earliest members of the group:

- Jaw joint - The dentary (the lower jaw bone which carries the teeth) and the squamosal (another small skull bone) meet to form the joint. In most gnathostomes, including early therapsids, the joint consists of the articular (a small bone at the back of the lower jaw) and the quadrate (a small bone at the back of the upper jaw).
- Middle ear - In crown-group mammals, sound is carried from the eardrum by a chain of three bones, the malleus,

the incus, and the stapes. Ancestrally, the malleus and the incus are derived from the articular and the quadrate bones that constituted the jaw joint of early therapsids.

- Tooth replacement - Teeth are replaced once or (as in toothed whales and murid rodents) not at all, rather than being replaced continually throughout life.
- Prismatic enamel - The enamel coating on the surface of a tooth consists of prisms, solid, rod-like structures extending from the dentin to the tooth's surface.
- Occipital condyles - Two knobs at the base of the skull fit into the topmost neck vertebra; most tetrapods, in contrast, have only one such knob.

For the most part, these characteristics were not present in the Triassic ancestors of the mammals. For palaeontologists who define Mammalia phylogenetically, no limit can be set on the features used to distinguish the group. Any feature may be relevant to a fossil's phylogenetic position. Palaeontologists defining Mammalia in terms of traits, on the other hand, need only consider those features that appear in the definition. The dentary-squamosal jaw joint is generally included.

Classification

George Gaylord Simpson's "Principles of Classification and a Classification of Mammals" (AMNH *Bulletin* v. 85, 1945) was the original source for the taxonomy listed here. Simpson laid out a systematics of mammal origins and relationships that was universally taught until the end of the 20th century. Since Simpson's classification, the paleontological record has been recalibrated, and the intervening years have seen much debate and progress concerning the theoretical underpinnings of systematization itself, partly through the new concept of cladistics. Though field work gradually made Simpson's classification outdated, it remained the closest thing to an official classification of mammals.

McKenna/Bell Classification

In 1997, the mammals were comprehensively revised by Malcolm C. McKenna and Susan K. Bell, which has resulted in the McKenna/Bell classification. Their 1997 book, *Classification of Mammals above the Species Level*, is the most comprehensive work to date on the systematics, relationships, and occurrences of all mammal taxa, living and extinct, down through the rank of genus, though recent molecular genetic data challenge several of the higher level groupings. The authors worked together as paleontologists at the American Museum of Natural History, New York. McKenna inherited the project from Simpson and, with Bell, constructed a completely updated hierarchical system, covering living and extinct taxa that reflects the historical genealogy of Mammalia.

The McKenna/Bell hierarchical listing of many terms used for mammal groups above the species includes extinct mammals, as well as modern groups, and introduces some fine distinctions such as legions and sublegions (ranks which fall between classes and orders) that are likely to be glossed over by the nonprofessionals.

Extinct groups are represented by a dagger (†).

Class Mammalia

- Subclass Prototheria: monotremes: echidnas and the platypus
- Subclass Theriiformes: live-bearing mammals and their prehistoric relatives.
    - Infraclass †Allotheria: multituberculates
    - Infraclass †Triconodonta: triconodonts
    - Infraclass Holotheria: modern live-bearing mammals and their prehistoric relatives.
        - Supercohort Theria: live-bearing mammals
        - Cohort Marsupialia: marsupials
        - Magnorder Australidelphia: Australian marsupials and the monito del monte
        - Magnorder Ameridelphia: New World marsupials.
        - Cohort Placentalia: placentals
        - Magnorder Xenarthra: xenarthrans
        - Magnorder Epitheria: epitheres
        - Grandorder Anagalida: lagomorphs, rodents, and elephant shrews

- Grandorder Ferae: carnivorans, pangolins, †creodonts, and relatives
- Grandorder Lipotyphla: insectivorans
- Grandorder Archonta: bats, primates, colugos, and treeshrews
- Grandorder Ungulata: ungulates
- Order Tubulidentata *incertae sedis*: aardvark
- Mirorder Eparctocyona: †condylarths, whales, and artiodactyls (even-toed ungulates)
- Mirorder †Meridiungulata: South American ungulates
- Mirorder Altungulata: perissodactyls (odd-toed ungulates), elephants, manatees, and hyraxes.

Molecular Classification of Placentals

Molecular studies based on DNA analysis have suggested new relationships among mammal families over the last few years. Most of these findings have been independently validated by retrotransposon presence/absence data. The most recent classification systems based on molecular studies have proposed four groups or lineages of placental mammals. Molecular clocks suggest that these clades diverged from early common ancestors in the Cretaceous, but fossils have not yet been found to corroborate this hypothesis. These molecular findings are consistent with mammal zoogeography:

Following molecular DNA sequence analyses, the first divergence was that of the Afrotheria 110–100 million years ago (mya). The Afrotheria proceeded to evolve and diversify in the isolation of the African-Arabian continent. The Xenarthra, isolated in South America, diverged from the Boreoeutheria approximately 100–95 million years ago. According to an alternative view, the Xenarthra has the Afrotheria as closest allies, forming the Atlantogenata as sister group to Boreoeutheria. The Boreoeutheria split into the Laurasiatheria and Euarchontoglires between 95 and 85 mya; both of these groups evolved on the northern continent of Laurasia. After tens of millions of years of relative isolation, Africa-Arabia collided with Eurasia, exchanging Afrotheria and Boreoeutheria.

The formation of the Isthmus of Panama linked South America and North America, which facilitated the exchange of mammal species in the Great American Interchange. The traditional view that no placental mammals reached Australasia until about 5 million years ago, when bats and murine rodents arrived, has been challenged by recent evidence and may need to be reassessed.

These molecular results are still controversial because they are not reflected by morphological data and therefore not accepted by many systematists. Further, there is some indication from retrotransposon presence/absence data that the traditional Epitheria hypothesis, suggesting Xenarthra as the first divergence, might be true.

With the old order Insectivora shown to be polyphylectic and more properly subdivided (as Afrosoricida, Erinaceomorpha, and Soricomorpha), the following classification for placental mammals contains 21 orders:

- Clade Atlantogenata
  - *Group I:* Afrotheria
    - Clade Afroinsectiphilia
    - *Order Macroscelidea:* elephant shrews (Africa)
    - *Order Afrosoricida:* tenrecs and golden moles (Africa)
    - *Order Tubulidentata:* aardvark (Africa south of the Sahara)
    - Clade Paenungulata
    - *Order Hyracoidea:* hyraxes or dassies (Africa, Arabia)
    - Order Proboscidea: elephants (Africa, Southeast Asia)
    - *Order Sirenia:* dugong and manatees (cosmopolitan tropical)
  - Group II: Xenarthra
    - *Order Pilosa:* sloths and anteaters (neotropical)
    - *Order Cingulata:* armadillos (Americas)

- Clade Boreoeutheria
  - *Group III:* Euarchontoglires (Supraprimates)
    - Superorder Euarchonta
    - *Order Scandentia:* treeshrews (Southeast Asia).
    - *Order Dermoptera:* flying lemurs or colugos (Southeast Asia)
    - *Order Primates:* lemurs, bushbabies, monkeys, apes, human (cosmopolitan)
    - Superorder Glires
    - *Order Lagomorpha:* pikas, rabbits, hares (Eurasia, Africa, Americas)
    - *Order Rodentia:* rodents (cosmopolitan)
  - *Group IV:* Laurasiatheria
    - *Order Erinaceomorpha:* hedgehogs
    - Order Soricomorpha: moles, shrews, solenodons
    - Clade Ferungulata
    - Clade Cetartiodactyla
    - *Order Cetacea:* whales, dolphins and porpoises
    - *Order Artiodactyla:* even-toed ungulates, including pigs, hippopotamus, camels, giraffe, deer, antelope, cattle, sheep, goats
    - Clade Pegasoferae
    - *Order Chiroptera:* bats (cosmopolitan)
    - Clade Zooamata
    - *Order Perissodactyla:* odd-toed ungulates, including horses, donkeys, zebras, tapirs, and rhinoceroses
    - Clade Ferae
    - *Order Pholidota:* pangolins or scaly anteaters (Africa, South Asia)
    - *Order Carnivora:* carnivores (cosmopolitan), including cats and dogs

- Synapsida, the group which contains mammals and their extinct relatives, originated during the Pennsylvanian subperiod, when they split from the lineage that led to reptiles and birds. Crown group mammals evolved from earlier mammaliaforms during the Early Jurassic.

Evolution from Amniotes in the Paleozoic

The first fully terrestrial vertebrates were amniotes. Like their amphibian predecessors, they have lungs and limbs. Amniotes' eggs, however, have internal membranes which allow the developing embryo to breathe but keep water in. Hence, amniotes can lay eggs on dry land, while amphibians generally need to lay their eggs in water.

The first amniotes apparently arose in the Late Carboniferous. They descended from earlier reptiliomorph amphibians, which lived on land already inhabited by insects and other invertebrates, and by ferns, mosses and other plants. Within a few million years, two important amniote lineages became distinct: the synapsids, which include mammals; and the sauropsids, which include turtles, lizards, snakes, crocodilians, dinosaurs and birds. Synapsids have a single hole (temporal fenestra) low on each side of the skull.

One synapsid group, the pelycosaurs, included the largest and fiercest animals of the early Permian. Therapsids descended from pelycosaurs in the middle Permian, about 265 million years ago, and took over their position as the dominant land vertebrates. They differ from pelycosaurs in several features of the skull and jaws, including: larger temporal fenestrae and incisors which are equal in size. The therapsid lineage leading to mammals went through a series of stages, beginning with animals that were very like their pelycosaur ancestors and ending with probainognathian cynodonts, some of which could easily be mistaken for mammals. Those stages were characterized by:

- gradual development of a bony secondary palate.
- Progress was made towards an erect limb posture, which would increase the animals' stamina by avoiding Carrier's constraint. But this process was slow and erratic: for example, all herbivorous nonmammaliaform

therapsids retained sprawling limbs (some late forms may have had semierect hind limbs); Permian carnivorous therapsids had sprawling forelimbs, and some late Permian ones also had semisprawling hindlimbs. In fact, modern monotremes still have semisprawling limbs.

- The dentary gradually became the main bone of the lower jaw and, in the Triassic, progressed towards the fully mammalian jaw (the lower consisting only of the dentary) and middle ear (which is constructed by the bones that were previously used to construct the jaws of reptiles).
- There is some evidence of hair in Triassic therapsids but none for Permian therapsids.
- Some Triassic therapsids also show signs of lactation. These nonmammalian synapsids are sometimes called "mammal-like reptiles".

The Mammals Appear

The Permian–Triassic extinction event, which was a prolonged event due to the accumulation of several extinction pulses, ended the dominance of the carnivores among the therapsids. In the early Triassic, all the medium to large land carnivore niches were taken over by archosaurs which, over an extended period of time (35 million years), came to include the crocodylomorphs, the pterosaurs, and the dinosaurs. By the Jurassic, the dinosaurs had come to dominate the large terrestrial herbivore niches as well. The first mammals (in the sense given to the term by Kielan-Jawarowska *et al.*) appeared in the Late Triassic epoch (about 210 million years ago), 60 million years after the first therapsids. They expanded out of their nocturnal insectivore niche from the mid-Jurassic onwards; *Castorocauda*, for example, had adaptations for swimming, digging and catching fish.

The majority of the mammal species that existed in the Mesozoic Era were multituberculates, triconodonts and spalacotheriids. The earliest known monotreme is *Teinolophos*, which lived about 123 million years ago in Australia. Monotremes have some features which may be inherited from the original amniotes:

- They use the same orifice to urinate, defecate and reproduce ("monotreme" means "one hole") – as lizards and birds also do.
- They lay eggs which are leathery and uncalcified, like those of lizards, turtles and crocodilians.

Unlike other mammals, female monotremes do not have nipples and feed their young by "sweating" milk from patches on their bellies. The earliest known metatherian is *Sinodelphys*, found in 125 million-year-old Early Cretaceous shale in China's northeastern Liaoning Province. The fossil is nearly complete and includes tufts of fur and imprints of soft tissues.

The oldest known fossil among the Eutheria ("true beasts") is the small shrewlike *Juramaia sinensis*, or "Jurassic mother from China," dated to 160 million years ago in the Upper Jurassic. A later eutherian, *Eomaia*, dated to 125 million years ago in the Lower Cretaceous, possessed some features in common with the marsupials but not with the placentals, evidence that these features were present in the last common ancestor of the two groups but were later lost in the placental lineage. In particular:

- Epipubic bones extend forwards from the pelvis. These are not found in any modern placental, but they are found in marsupials, monotremes, and nontherian mammals like the multituberculates as well as in *Ukhaatherium*, an Upper Cretaceous animal in the eutherian order Asioryctitheria. They are apparently an ancestral feature which subsequently disappeared in the placental lineage. These epipubic bones seem to function by stiffening the muscles of these animals during locomotion, reducing the amount of space being presented, which placentals require to contain their fetus during gestation periods.
- A narrow pelvic outlet indicates that the young were very small at birth and therefore pregnancy was short, as in modern marsupials. This suggests that the placenta was a later development.

When true placental mammals evolved is uncertain – the earliest undisputed fossils of placentals come from the early Paleocene, after the extinction of the dinosaurs.

Rise to Dominance in the Cenozoic

Mammals took over the medium- to large-sized ecological niches in the Cenozoic, after the Cretaceous–Paleogene extinction event emptied ecological space once filled by reptiles. Then mammals diversified very quickly; both birds and mammals show an exponential rise in diversity. For example, the earliest known bat dates from about 50 million years ago, only 15 million years after the extinction of the dinosaurs.

Recent molecular phylogenetic studies suggest that most placental orders diverged about 100 to 85 million years ago and that modern families appeared in the period from the late Eocene through the Miocene. But paleontologists object that no placental fossils have been found from before the end of the Cretaceous. During the Cenozoic, several groups of mammals appeared which were much larger than their nearest modern equivalents, but none was even close to the size of the largest dinosaurs with similar feeding habits.

Earliest Appearances of Features

Hadrocodium, whose fossils date from the early Jurassic (approximately 195 million years ago, in the Lower Jurassic), provides the first clear evidence of a jaw joint formed solely by the squamosal and dentary bones; there is no space in the jaw for the articular, a bone involved in the jaws of all early synapsids. It has been suggested that the original function of lactation (milk production) was to keep eggs moist. Much of the argument is based on monotremes (egg-laying mammals).

The earliest clear evidence of hair or fur is in fossils of *Castorocauda*, from 164 million years ago in the Middle Jurassic. In the past, some scientists interpreted the foramina (passages) in the maxillae (upper jaws) and premaxillae (small bones in front of the maxillae) of cynodonts as channels which supplied blood vessels and nerves to vibrissae (whiskers) and suggested that this was evidence of hair or fur. Foramina do not necessarily show that an animal had vibrissae, however; the modern lizard *Tupinambis* has foramina which are almost identical to those found in the nonmammalian cynodont Thrinaxodon. The evolution of erect limbs in mammals is incomplete — living and fossil monotremes have sprawling limbs. The parasagittal (nonsprawling) limb posture appeared sometime in the Early

Cretaceous or latest Jurassic; it is found in the eutherian *Eomaia* and the metatherian *Sinodelphys*, both dated 125 million years ago.

When endothermy first appeared in the evolution of mammals is uncertain. Modern monotremes have lower body temperatures and more variable metabolic rates than marsupials and placentals, but there is evidence that some of their ancestors, perhaps including ancestors of the therians, may have had body temperatures like those of modern therians. Some of the evidence found so far suggests that Triassic cynodonts had fairly high metabolic rates, but it is not conclusive. For small animals, an insulative covering like fur is necessary for the maintenance of a high and stable body temperature.

Anatomy and Morphology

Skeletal System: The majority of mammals have seven cervical vertebrae (bones in the neck), including bats, giraffes, whales, and humans. The exceptions are the manatee and the two-toed sloth, which have only six cervical vertebrae, and the three-toed sloth with nine cervical vertebrae.

Respiratory System: The lungs of mammals have a spongy texture and are honeycombed with epithelium having a much larger surface area in total than the outer surface area of the lung itself. The lungs of humans are typical of this type of lung.

Breathing is largely driven by the muscular diaphragm, which divides the thorax from the abdominal cavity, forming a dome with its convexity towards the thorax. Contraction of the diaphragm flattens the dome, increasing the volume of the cavity in which the lung is enclosed. Air enters through the oral and nasal cavities; it flows through the larynx, trachea and bronchi and expands the alveoli. Relaxation of the diaphragm has the opposite effect, passively recoiling during normal breathing. During exercise, the abdominal wall contracts, increasing visceral pressure on the diaphragm, thus forcing the air out more quickly and forcefully. The rib cage itself also is able to expand and contract the thoracic cavity to some degree, through the action of other respiratory and accessory respiratory muscles. As a result, air is sucked into or expelled out of the lungs, always moving down its pressure gradient. This type of lung is known as a bellows lung as it resembles a blacksmith's bellows. Mammals take oxygen into their lungs, and discard carbon dioxide.

Nervous System: All mammalian brains possess a neocortex, a brain region unique to mammals. Placental mammals have a corpus callosum, unlike monotremes and marsupials. The size and number of cortical areas (Brodmann's areas) is least in monotremes (about 8-10) and most in placentals (up to 50).

Integumentary System: The integumentary system is made up of three layers: the outermost epidermis, the dermis, and the hypodermis. The epidermis is typically 10 to 30 cells thick; its main function is to provide a waterproof layer. Its outermost cells are constantly lost; its bottommost cells are constantly dividing and pushing upward.

The middle layer, the dermis, is 15 to 40 times thicker than the epidermis. The dermis is made up of many components, such as bony structures and blood vessels. The hypodermis is made up of adipose tissue. Its job is to store lipids, and to provide cushioning and insulation. The thickness of this layer varies widely from species to species. Although other animals have features such as feathers, whiskers, setae, or cilia that superficially resemble it, no animals other than mammals have hair. It is a definitive characteristic of the class. Though some mammals have very little, careful examination reveals the characteristic, often in obscure parts of their bodies. Some primates and marsupials have shades of violet, green, or blue skin on parts of their bodies. The two-toed sloth and the polar bear sometimes appear to have green fur, but this colour is caused by algae growths.

Reproductive System

Most mammals are viviparous, giving birth to live young. However, the five species of monotreme, the platypuses and the echidnas, lay eggs. The monotremes have a sex determination system different from that of most other mammals. In particular, the sex chromosomes of a platypus are more like those of a chicken than those of a therian mammal. The mammary glands of mammals are specialised to produce milk, a liquid used by newborns as their primary source of nutrition. The monotremes branched early from other mammals and do not have the nipples seen in most mammals, but they do have mammary glands. The young lick the milk from a mammary patch on the mother's belly. Viviparous mammals are in the subclass Theria; those living today are in the marsupial and placental infraclasses. A marsupial has a short gestation period, typically shorter than its estrous cycle, and gives birth to an undeveloped newborn that then undergoes further development; in many species, this takes place within a pouch-like sac, the marsupium, located in the front of the mother's abdomen. The placentals give birth to complete and fully developed young, usually after long gestation periods.

Physiology

Endothermy: Nearly all mammals are endothermic ("warm-blooded"). Most mammals also have hair to help keep them warm. Like birds, mammals can forage or hunt in weather and climates too cold for nonavian reptiles and large insects.

Endothermy requires plenty of food energy, so mammals eat more food per unit of body weight than most reptiles. Small insectivorous mammals eat prodigious amounts for their size.

A rare exception, the naked mole rat, produces little metabolic heat, so it is considered an operational poikilotherm. Birds are also endothermic, so endothermy is not a defining mammalian feature.

Intelligence

In intelligent mammals, such as primates, the cerebrum is larger relative to the rest of the brain. Intelligence itself is not easy to define, but indications of intelligence include the ability to learn, matched with behavioural flexibility.

Rats, for example, are considered to be highly intelligent, as they can learn and perform new tasks, an ability that may be important when they first colonize a fresh habitat. In some mammals, food gathering appears to be related to intelligence: a deer feeding on plants has a brain smaller than a cat, which must think to outwit its prey.

Animal Locomotion

Animal locomotion, which is the act of self-propulsion by an animal, has many manifestations, including running, swimming, jumping and flying. Animals move for a variety of reasons, such as to find food, a mate, or a suitable microhabitat, and to escape predators. For many animals the ability to move is essential to survival and, as a result, selective pressures have shaped the locomotion methods and mechanisms employed by moving organisms.

For example, migratory animals that travel vast distances (such as the Arctic Tern) typically have a locomotion mechanism that costs very little energy per unit distance, whereas non-migratory animals that must frequently move quickly to escape predators (such as frogs) are likely to have costly but very fast locomotion. The study of animal locomotion is typically considered to be a sub-field of biomechanics.

Locomotion requires energy to overcome friction, drag, inertia, and gravity, though in many circumstances some of these factors are negligible. In terrestrial environments gravity must be overcome, though the drag of air is much less of an issue. In aqueous environments however, friction (or drag) becomes the major challenge, with gravity being less of a concern.

Although animals with natural buoyancy need not expend much energy maintaining vertical position, some will naturally sink and must expend energy to remain afloat. Drag may also present a problem in flight, and the aerodynamically efficient body shapes of birds highlight this point.

Flight presents a different problem from movement in water however, as there is no way for a living organism to have lower density than air. Limbless organisms moving on land must often contend with surface friction, but do not usually need to expend significant energy to counteract gravity. Newton's third law of motion is widely used in the study of animal locomotion: if at rest, to move forwards an animal must push something backwards.

Terrestrial animals must push the solid ground, swimming and flying animals must push against a fluid or gas (either water or air). The effect of forces during locomotion on the design of the skeletal system is also important, as is the interaction between locomotion and muscle physiology, in determining how the structures and effectors of locomotion enable or limit animal movement.

Introduction

Animals move through a variety of fluids, such as water, air and mud. Some, for example seals and otters, move through more than one type of fluid. In some cases locomotion is facilitated by the substrate on which they move. Forms of locomotion include:

Through a Fluid Medium

Swimming: In the water staying afloat is possible through buoyancy. Provided an aquatic animal's body is no denser than its aqueous environment, it should be able to stay afloat well enough. Though this means little energy need be expended maintaining vertical position, it makes movement in the horizontal plane much more difficult.

The drag encountered in water is much higher than that of air, which is almost negligible at low speeds. Body shape is therefore important for efficient movement, which is essential for basic functions like catching prey. A fusiform, torpedo-like body form is seen in many marine animals, though the mechanisms they employ for movement are diverse. Movement of the body may be from side to side, as in sharks and many fishes, or up and down, as in marine mammals.

Other animals, such as those from the class *Cephalopoda*, use jet-propulsion, taking in water then squirting it back out in an explosive burst. Others may rely predominantly on their limbs, much as humans do when swimming. Though life on land originated from the seas, terrestrial animals have returned to an aquatic lifestyle on several occasions, such as the fully aquatic cetaceans, now far removed from their terrestrial ancestors.

Flight

Gravity is the primary obstacle to flight through the air. Because it is impossible for any organism to have a density as low as that of air, flying animals must generate enough lift to ascend and remain airborne. Wing shape is crucial in achieving this, generating a pressure gradient that results in an upward force on the animal's body.

The same principle applies to airplanes, the wings of which are also airfoils. Unlike aircraft however, flying animals must be very light to achieve flight, the largest living flying animals being birds of around 20 kilograms. Other structural modifications of flying animals include reduced and redistributed body weight, fusiform shape and powerful flight muscles.

Rather than fly, some animals simply reduce their rate of falling by gliding. Flight has independently evolved at least four times, in the insects, pterosaurs, birds, and bats. Gliding has evolved on many more occasions.

On a Substrate

Terrestrial: Forms of locomotion on land include walking, running, hopping or jumping, and crawling or slithering. Here friction and buoyancy are no longer an issue, but a strong skeletal and muscular framework are required in most terrestrial animals for structural support. Each step also requires much energy to overcome inertia, and animals can store elastic potential energy in their tendons to help overcome this. Balance is also required for movement on land. Human infants learn to crawl first before they are able to stand on two feet, which requires good coordination as well as physical development. Humans are bipedal animals, standing on two feet and keeping one on the ground at all times while walking. When running, only one foot is on the ground at any one time at most, and both leave the ground briefly.

At higher speeds momentum helps keep the body upright, so more energy can be used in movement. The number of legs an animal has varies greatly, resulting in differences in locomotion. Many familiar mammals have four legs; insects have six, while arachnids have eight. Centipedes and millipedes have many sets of legs that move in metachronal rhythm. Some have none at all, relying on other modes of locomotion.

Other animals move in terrestrial habitats without the aid of legs. Earthworms crawl by a peristalsis, the same rhythmic contractions that propel food through the digestive tract. Snakes move using several different modes of locomotion, depending upon substrate type and desired speed. Some animals even roll, though typically not as a primary means of locomotion. Some animals are specialised for moving on non-horizontal surfaces. One common habitat for such climbing animals is in trees, for example the gibbon is specialised for arboreal movement, traveling rapidly by brachiation. Another case is animals like the snow leopard living on steep rock faces such as are found in mountains. Some light animals are able to climb up smooth sheer surfaces or hang upside down by adhesion. Many insects can do this, though much larger animals such as geckos can also perform similar feats.

On Water

While animals like ducks can swim in water by floating, some small animals move across it without breaking through the surface. This surface locomotion takes advantage of the surface tension of water.

Animals that move in such a way include the water strider. Water striders have legs that are hydrophobic, preventing them from interfering with the structure of water. Another form of locomotion (in which the surface layer is broken) is used by the Basilisk lizard.

Through a Solid Medium

Some animals move through solids such as soil by burrowing using claws, teeth, or other methods. A burrow is a hole or tunnel dug into the ground by an animal to create a space suitable for habitation, temporary refuge, or as a byproduct of locomotion. In loose solids such a sand some animals, such as the golden mole, marsupial mole, and the pink fairy armadillo, are able to move more rapidly, 'swimming' through the loose substrate. Burrowing animals include moles, ground squirrels, naked mole rats, tilefish, mole crickets, and earthworms.

Energetics

The energetics of locomotion involves the energy expenditure by animals in moving. Energy consumed in locomotion is not available for other efforts, so animals typically have evolved to use the minimum energy possible during movement. However, in the case of certain behaviours, such as locomotion to escape a predator, performance (such as speed or maneuverability) is more crucial, and such movements may be energetically expensive. Furthermore, animals may use energetically expensive methods of locomotion when environmental conditions (such as being within a tunnel) preclude other modes.

The most common metric of energy use during locomotion is net cost of transport, defined as the calories needed above baseline metabolism to move a given distance, per unit body mass. For aerobic locomotion, most animals have a nearly constant cost of transport - moving a given distance requires the same caloric expenditure, regardless of speed.

This constancy is usually accomplished by changes in gait. The net cost of transport of swimming is lowest, followed by flight, with terrestrial limbed locomotion being the most expensive per unit distance.

However, because of the speeds involved, flight requires the most energy per unit time. This does not mean that an animal that normally moves by running would be a more efficient swimmer, however; these comparisons assume an animal is specialised for that form of motion. Another consideration here is body mass—heavier animals, though using more total energy, require less energy *per unit mass* to move. Physiologists generally measure energy use by the amount of oxygen consumed, or the amount of carbon dioxide produced, in an animal's respiration.

Methods of Study

A variety of methods and equipment are used to study animal locomotion:

- Kinematics is the study of the motion of an entire animal or parts of its body. It is typically accomplished by placing visual markers at particular anatomical locations on the animal and then recording video of its movement. The video is often captured from multiple angles, with frame rates exceeding 2000 frames per second when capturing high speed movement. The location of each marker is determined for each video frame, and data from multiple views is integrated to give positions of each point through time. Computers are sometimes used to track the markers, although this task must often be performed manually. The kinematic data can be used to determine fundamental motion attributes such as velocity, acceleration, joint angles, and the sequencing and timing of kinematic events. These fundamental attributes can be used to quantify various higher level attributes, such as the physical abilities of the animal (e.g., its maximum running speed, how steep a slope it can climb), neural control of locomotion, gait, and responses to environmental variation. These, in turn, can aid in formulation of hypotheses about the animal or locomotion in general.

- Force plates are platforms, usually part of a trackway, that can be used to measure the magnitude and direction of forces of an animal's step. When used with kinematics and a sufficiently detailed model of anatomy, inverse dynamics solutions can determine the forces not just at the contact with the ground, but at each joint in the limb.
- Electromyography (EMG) is a method of detecting the electrical activity that occurs when muscles are activated, thus determining which muscles are used when in a given movement. This can be accomplished either by surface electrodes (usually in large animals) or implanted electrodes (often wires thinner than a human hair). Furthermore, the intensity of electrical activity can correlate to the level of muscle activity, with greater activity implying (though not definitively showing) greater force.
- Sonomicrometry employs a pair of piezoelectric crystals implanted in a muscle or tendon to continuously measure the length of a muscle or tendon. This is useful because surface kinematics may be inaccurate due to skin movement. Similarly, if an elastic tendon is in series with the muscle, the muscle length may not be accurately reflected by the joint angle.
- Tendon force buckles measure the force produced by a single muscle by measuring the strain of a tendon. After the experiment, the tendon's elastic modulus is determined and used to compute the exact force produced by the muscle. However, this can only be used on muscles with long tendons.
- Particle image velocimetry is used in aquatic and aerial systems to measure the flow of fluid around and past a moving aquatic organism, allowing fluid dynamics calculations to determine pressure gradients, speeds, etc.

- Fluoroscopy allows real-time X-ray video, for precise kinematics of moving bones. Markers which are opaque to X-rays can allow simultaneous tracking of muscle length.

All of the methods can be combined. For example, studies frequently combine EMG and kinematics to determine "motor pattern", the series of electrical and kinematic events which produce a given movement.

Terrestrial Locomotion

Terrestrial locomotion has evolved as animals adapted from aquatic to terrestrial environments. Locomotion on land raises different problems than that in water, with reduced friction being replaced by the effects of gravity. There are three basic forms of locomotion found among terrestrial animals

- *Legged* - Moving by using appendages
- *Limbless locomotion* - moving without legs, primarily using the body itself as a propulsive structure.
- *Rolling* - rotating the body over the substrate.

Legged Locomotion

Movement on appendages is the most common form of terrestrial locomotion, it is the basic form of locomotion of two major groups with many terrestrial members, the vertebrates and the arthropods. Important aspects of legged locomotion are posture (the way the body is supported by the legs), the number of legs, and the functional structure of the leg and foot. There are also many gaits, ways of moving the legs to locomote, such as walking, running, or jumping.

Posture

Appendages can be used for movement in a number of ways. The posture, the way the body is supported by the legs, is an important aspect. There are three main ways in which vertebrates support themselves with their legs - sprawling, semi-erect, and fully erect. Some animals may use different postures in different circumstances, depending on the posture's mechanical advantages. Interestingly, there is no detectable difference in energetic cost between stances. The "sprawling" posture is the most primitive, and is the original limb posture from which the others evolved. The upper limbs are typically held horizontally, while the lower limbs are vertical, though upper limb angle may be substantially increased in large animals. The body may drag along the ground, as in salamanders, or may be substantially elevated, as in monitor lizards. This posture is typically associated with trotting gaits, and the body flexes from side-to-side during movement to increase step length.

All limbed reptiles and salamanders use this posture, as does the platypus and several species of frogs that walk. Unusual examples can be founds among amphibious fish, such as the mudskipper, which drag themselves across land on their sturdy fins. Among the invertebrates, most arthropods—which includes the most diverse group of animals, the insects—have a stance best described as sprawling. There is also anecdotal evidence that some octopus species (such as the *Pinnoctopus* genus) can also drag themselves across land a short distance by hauling their body along by their tentacles (for example to pursue prey between rockpools) - there may be video evidence of this. The semi-erect posture is more accurately interpreted as an extremely elevated sprawling posture. This mode of locomotion is typically found in large lizards such as monitor lizards and tegus.

Mammals and birds typically have a fully erect posture, though each evolved it independently. In these groups the legs are placed beneath the body. This is often linked with the evolution of endothermy, as it avoids Carrier's constraint and thus allows prolonged periods of activity (Bakker 1988).

The fully erect stance is not necessarily the "most-evolved" stance; evidence suggests that crocodilians evolved a semi-erect stance in their forelimbs from ancestors with fully erect stance as a result of adapting to a mostly aquatic lifestyle, though their hindlimbs are still held fully erect. For example, the mesozoic prehistoric crocodilian *Erpetosuchus* is believed to have had a fully erect stance and been terrestrial.

Number of Legs

The number of locomotory appendages varies much between animals, and sometimes the same animal may use different numbers of its legs in different circumstances. The best contender for unipedal movement is the springtail, which while normally hexapedal, hurls itself away from danger using its furcula, a tail-like forked rod that can be rapidly unfurled from the underside of its body. A number of species move and stand on two legs, that is, they are bipedal. The group that is exclusively bipedal is the birds, which have either an alternating or a hopping gait. There are also a number of bipedal mammals. Most of these move by hopping – including the macropods such as kangaroos and various jumping rodents. Only a few mammals such as humans and the ground pangolin commonly show an alternating bipedal gait. Also cockroaches and some lizards may run on their two hind legs.

With the exception of the birds, all terrestrial vertebrate groups with legs are mostly quadrupedal – the mammals, reptiles, and the amphibians usually move on four legs. There are many quadrupedal gaits. The most diverse group of animals on earth, the insects, are included in a larger taxon known as hexapods, most of which are hexapedal, walking and standing on six legs. Exceptions among the insects include praying mantises and water scorpions, which are quadrupeds with their front two legs modified for grasping, some butterflies which use only four legs, and some kinds of insect larvae that may have no legs (e.g., maggots), or additional prolegs (e.g., caterpillars). Spiders and many of their relatives move on eight legs – they are octopedal. However, some creatures move on many more legs. Terrestrial crustaceans may have a fair number - woodlice having fourteen legs. Also, as previously mentioned, some insect larvae such as caterpillars and sawfly larvae have up to five (caterpillars) or nine (sawflies) additional fleshy prolegs in addition to the six legs normal for insects.

Some species of invertebrate have even more legs, the unusual velvet worm having stubby legs under the length of its body, with around several dozen pairs of legs. Centipedes have one pair of legs per body segment, with typically around 50 legs, but some species have over 200. The terrestrial animals with the most legs are the millipedes. They have two pairs of legs per body segment, with common species having between 80 and 400 legs overall – with the rare species *Illacme plenipes* having up to 750 legs. Animals with many legs typically move them in metachronal rhythm, which gives the appearance of waves of motion travelling forwards along their rows of legs.

Leg and Foot Structure

The legs of tetrapods, the main group of terrestrial vertebrates, have internal bones, with externally attached muscles for movement, and the basic form has three key joints: the shoulder joint, the knee joint, and the ankle joint, at which the foot is attached. Within this theme there is much variation in form. An alternative form of vertebrate 'leg' to the tetrapod leg is the fins found on amphibious fish. Also a few tetrapods, such as the macropods, have adapted their tails as additional locomotory appendages.

The basic form of the vertebrate foot has five toes, however some animals will have evolved fewer than this, and some early tetrapods had more; Acanthostega had eight toes. Feet have evolved many forms depending on the animal's needs. One key variation is where on the foot the animal's weight is placed. Most vertebrates—the amphibians, the reptiles, and some mammals such as humans and bears—are plantigrade, walking on the whole of the underside of the foot.

Many mammals, such as cats and dogs are digitigrade, walking on their toes, the greater stride length allowing more speed. Digitigrade mammals are also often adept at quiet movement. Birds are also digitigrade. Some animals such as horses are unguligrade, walking on the tips of their toes. This even further increases their stride length and thus their speed. A few mammals are also known to walk on their knuckles, at least for their front legs. Knuckle-walking allows the foot (hand) to specialise for food gathering and/or climbing, as with the great apes and the extinct chalicotheres, or for swimming, as with the platypus. In animals where feet have evolved into functional hands, hand walking is also possible.

Among terrestrial invertebrates there are a number of leg forms. The arthropod legs are jointed and supported by hard external armor, with the muscles attached to the internal surface of this exoskeleton. The other group of legged terrestrial invertebrates, the velvet worms, have soft stumpy legs supported by a hydrostatic skeleton. The prolegs that some caterpillars have in addition to their six more-standard arthropod legs have a similar form to those of velvet worms, and suggest a distant shared ancestry.

Gaits

Animals show a vast range of gaits, the order that they place and lift their appendages in locomotion. Gaits can be grouped into categories according to their patterns of support sequence. For quadrupeds, there are three main categories: walking gaits, running gaits, and leaping gaits. In one system, there are 60 discrete patterns: 37 walking gaits, 14 running gaits, and 9 leaping gaits. Walking is the most common gait, where some feet are on the ground at any given time, and found in almost all legged animals. In an informal sense, running is considered to occur when at some points in the stride all feet are off the ground in a moment of suspension.

Technically, however, moments of suspension occur in both running gaits (such as trot) and leaping gaits (such as canter and gallop). Gaits involving one or more moments of suspension can be found in many animals, and compared to walking they are faster but more energetically costly forms of locomotion.

Animals will use different gaits for different speeds, terrain, and situations. For example horses show four natural gaits, the slowest horse gait is the walk, then there are three faster gaits which, from slowest to fastest, are the trot, the canter, and the gallop. Animals may also have unusual gaits that are used occasionally, such as for moving sideways or backwards. For example, the main human gaits are bipedal walking and running, but they employ many other gaits occasionally, including a four-legged crawl in tight spaces.

In walking, and for many animals running, the motion of legs on either side of the body alternates, i.e. is out of phase. Other animals, such as a horse when galloping, or an inchworm, alternate between their front and back legs. An alternative to a gait that alternates between legs is hopping or saltation, where all legs move together. As a main means of locomotion, this is usually found in bipeds or semi-bipeds.

Among the mammals saltation is commonly used among macropods (kangaroos and their relatives), jerboas, springhares, kangaroo rats, hopping mice, gerbils, and sportive lemurs. Certain tendons in kangaroo hind legs are very elastic, allowing kangaroos to effectively bounce along conserving energy from hop to hop, making hopping a very energy efficient way to move around in their nutrient poor environment. Saltation is also used by many small birds. Frogs and fleas also hop.

Most animals move in the direction of their head. However there are some exceptions. Crabs move sideways, and naked mole rats, which live in tight tunnels underground, can move backward or forward with equal facility. Crayfish can move backward much faster than they can move forward. Gait analysis is the study of gait in humans and other animals. This may involve videoing subjects with markers on particular anatomical landmarks and measuring the forces of their footfall using floor transducers (strain gauges). Skin electrodes may also be used to measure muscle activity.

Limbless Locomotion

There are a number of terrestrial and amphibious limbless vertebrates and invertebrates. These animals, due to lack of appendages, use their bodies to generate propulsive force. These movements are sometimes referred to as "slithering" or "crawling", although neither are formally used in the scientific literature and the latter term is also used for some animals moving on all four limbs. All limbless animals come from cold-blooded groups; there are no endothermic limbless animals, i.e. there are no limbless birds or mammals.

Lower Body Surface

Where the foot is important to the legged mammal, for limbless animals the underside of the body is important. Some animals such as snakes or legless lizards move on their smooth dry underside. Other animals have various features that aid movement. Molluscs such as slugs and snails move on a layer of mucus that is secreted from their underside, reducing friction and protecting from injury when moving over sharp objects. Earthworms have small bristles (setae) that hook into the substrate and help them move. Some animals such as leeches have suction cups on either end of the body allowing two anchor movement.

Type of Movement

Some limbless animals, such as leeches, have suction cups on either end of their body, which allow them to move by anchoring the rear end and then moving forward the front end, which is then anchored and then the back end is pulled in, and so on. This is known as two-anchor movement. A legged animal, the inchworm, also moves like this, clasping with appendages at either end of its body.

Limbless animals can also move using pedal locomotary waves, rippling the underside of the body. This is the main method used by molluscs such as slugs and snails, and also large flatworms, some other worms, and even earless seals. The waves may move in the opposite direction to motion, known as retrograde waves, or in the same direction as motion, known as direct waves. Earthworms move by retrograde waves alternatively swelling and contracting down the length of their body, the swollen sections being held in place using setae. Aquatic molluscs such as limpets, which are sometimes out of the water, tend to move using retrograde waves. However terrestrial molluscs such as slugs and snails tend to use direct waves. Lugworms and seals also use direct waves.

Most snakes move using lateral undulation where a lateral wave travels down the snake's body in the opposite direction to the snake's motion and pushes the snake off irregularities in the ground. This mode of locomotion requires these irregularities to function. Another form of locomotion, rectilinear locomotion, is used at times by some snakes, especially large ones such as pythons and boa.

Here large scales on the underside of the body, known as scutes are used to push backwards and downwards. This is effective on a flat surface and is used for slow, silent movement, such as when stalking prey. Snakes use concertina locomotion for moving slowly in tunnels, here the snake alternates in bracing parts of its body on it surrounds. Finally the caenophidian snakes use the fast and unusual method of movement known as sidewinding on sand or loose soil. The snake cycles through throwing the front part of its body in the direction of motion and bringing the back part of its body into line crosswise.

Rolling

Although animals have never evolved wheels for locomotion, a small number of animals will move at times by rolling their whole body. Rolling animals can be divided into those that roll under the force of gravity or wind and those that roll using their own power.

Gravity or Wind Assisted

Web-toed salamander. This 10 cm long salamander lives on steep hills in the Sierra Nevada mountains. When it's disturbed or startled it coils itself up into a little ball often causing it to roll down hill. Pebble toad (*Oreophrynella niger*). This toad lives atop tepui in the Guiana highlands of South America. When threatened, often by tarantulas, it rolls into ball, and typically being on an incline, rolls away under gravity like a loose pebble. Namib wheeling spiders (*Carparachne spp.*), found in the Namib desert, will actively roll down sand dunes. This action can be used to successfully escape predators such as the *Pompilidae* tarantula wasps, which lay their eggs in a paralyzed spider for their larvae to feed on when they hatch. The spiders flip their body sideways and then cartwheel over their bent legs. The rotation is fast, with the golden wheel Spider (*Carparachne aureoflava*) moving up to 20 revolutions per second, moving the spider at 1 metre per second. Coastal tiger beetle larvae when threatened can flick themselves into the air and curl their bodies to form a wheels, which the wind blows, often uphill, as far as 25m and as fast as 11kph. The also may have some ability to steer themselves in this state. Pangolins, a type of mammal covered in thick scales rolls into a tight ball when threatened. Pangolins has been reported to roll away from danger, by both gravity and self-powered methods. A pangolin in hill country in Sumatra, to flee from the researcher, ran to the edge of a slope and curled into a ball to roll down the slope, crashing through the vegetation, and covering an estimated 30 metres or more in 10 seconds.

Self-Powered

Caterpillar of the Mother-Of-Pearl Moth, Pleuroptya ruralis. When attacked, this caterpillar will touch its head to its tail and roll backwards, up to 5 revolutions at about 40 cm per second, which is about 40 times its normal speed. Nannosquilla decemspinosa, a species of long-bodied, short-legged Mantis Shrimp, lives in shallow sandy areas along the Pacific coast of Central and South America. When stranded by a low tide the 3 cm stomatopod lies on its back and performs backwards somersaults over and over. The animal moves up to 2 metres at a time by rolling 20-40 times, with speeds of around 72 revolutions per minute. That is 1.5 body lengths per second (3.5 cm/s). Researchers estimate that the stomatopod acts as a true wheel around 40% of the time during this series of rolls. The remaining 60% of the time it has to "jumpstart" a roll by using its body to thrust itself upwards and forwards. Pangolins have also been reported to roll away from danger by self-powered methods. Witnessed by a lion researcher in the Serengeti in Africa, a group of lions surrounded a pangolin, but could not get purchase on it when it rolled into a ball, and so the lions sat around it waiting and dozing. Surrounded by lions, it would unroll itself slightly and give itself a push to roll some distance, until by doing this multiple times it could get far enough away from the lions to be safe. Moving like this would allow a pangolin to cover distance while still remaining in a protective armoured ball .

Limits and Extremes: The fastest terrestrial animal is the cheetah, which can attain maximal sprint speeds of approximately 104 km/h (64 mph). The fastest running lizard is the Black Iguana, which has been recorded moving at speed of up to 34.9 km/h (21.7 mph).

Arboreal Locomotion

Arboreal locomotion is the locomotion of animals in trees. In every habitat in which trees are present, animals have evolved to move in them. Some animals may only scale trees occasionally, while others are exclusively arboreal. These habitats pose numerous mechanical challenges to animals moving through them, leading to a variety of anatomical, behavioural and ecological consequences. Furthermore, many of these same principles may be applied to climbing without trees, such as on rock piles or mountains. The earliest known tetrapod with specialisations that adapted it for climbing trees, was *Suminia*, a synapsid of the late Permian, about 260 million years ago. Some invertebrate animals are exclusively arboreal in habitat.

Biomechanics: Arboreal habitats pose numerous mechanical challenges to animals moving in them, which have been solved diverse ways. These challenges include moving on narrow branches, moving up and down inclines, balancing, crossing gaps, and dealing with obstructions

Diametre: Moving along a narrow surface poses special difficulties to animals. During locomotion on the ground, the location of the centre of mass may swing from side to side, but during arboreal locomotion, this would result in the centre of mass moving beyond the edge of the branch, resulting in a tendency to topple over. Additionally, foot placement is constrained by the need to make contact with the narrow branch. This narrowness severely restricts the range of movements and postures an animal can use to move.

Incline: Branches are frequently oriented at an angle to gravity in arboreal habitats, including being vertical, which poses special problems. As an animal moves up an inclined branch, they must fight the force of gravity to raise their body, making movement more difficult. Conversely, as the animal descends, it must also fight gravity to control its descent and prevent falling. Descent can be particularly problematic for many animals, and highly arboreal species often have specialised methods for controlling their descent.

Balance: Due to the height of many branches and the potentially disastrous consequences of a fall, balance is of primary importance to arboreal animals. On horizontal and gently sloped branches, the primary problem is tipping to the side due to the narrow base of support. The narrower the branch, the greater the difficulty in balancing a given animal faces. On steep and vertical branches, tipping becomes less of an issue, and pitching backwards or slipping downwards becomes the most likely failure. In this case, large-diametre branches pose a greater challenge, since the animal cannot place its forelimbs closer to the centre of the branch than its hindlimbs.

Crossing Gaps: Branches are not continuous, and any arboreal animal must be able to move between gaps in the branches, or even between trees. This can be accomplished by reaching across gaps, or by leaping across them.

Obstructions: Arboreal habitats often contain many obstructions, both in the form of branches emerging from the one being moved on and other branches impinging on the space the animal needs to move through. These obstructions may impede locomotion, or may be used as additional contact points to enhance it, but only one laboratory study has ever quantified the results of obstructions.

Anatomical Specialisations: Arboreal organisms display many specialisations for dealing with the mechanical challenges of moving through their habitats.

Limb Length: Arboreal animals frequently have elongated limbs that help them cross gaps, reach fruit or other resources, test the firmness of support ahead, and in some cases, to brachiate. However, some species of lizard have reduced limb size that helps them avoid limb movement being obstructed by impinging branches.

Prehensile Tails: Many arboreal species, such as tree porcupines, chameleons, Silky Anteaters, spider monkeys, and possums, use prehensile tails to grasp branches. In the spider monkey and crested gecko, the tip of the tail has either a bare patch or adhesive pad, which provide increased friction.

Claws: Claws can be used to interact with rough substrates and re-orient the direction of forces the animal applies. This is what allows squirrels to climb tree trunks that are so large as to be essentially flat, from the perspective of such a small animal. However, claws can interfere with an animal's ability to grasp very small branches, as they may wrap too far around and prick the animal's own paw.

Adhesion: Adhesion is an alternative to claws, which works best on smooth surfaces. Wet adhesion is common in tree frogs and arboreal salamanders, and functions either by suction or by capilary adhesion. Dry adhesion is best typified by the specialised toes of geckos, which use van der Waals forces to adhere to many substrates, even glass.

Gripping: Frictional gripping is used by primates, relying upon hairless fingertips. Squeezing the branch between the fingertips generates frictional force that holds the animal's hand to the branch.

However, this type of grip depends upon the angle of the frictional force, thus upon the diametre of the branch, with larger branches resulting in reduced gripping ability. Animals other than primates that use gripping in climbing include the chameleon, which has mitten-like grasping feet, and many birds that grip branches in perching or moving about.

Reversible Feet: To control descent, especially down large diametre branches, some arboreal animals such as squirrels have evolved highly mobile ankle joints that permit rotating the foot into a 'reversed' posture. This allows the claws to hook into the rough surface of the bark, opposing the force of gravity.

Low Centre of Mass: Many arboreal species lower their centre of mass to reduce pitching and toppling movement when climbing. This may be accomplished by postural changes, altered body proportions, or smaller size.

Small Size: Small size provides many advantages to arboreal species, such as increasing the relative size of branches to the animal, lower centre of mass, increased stability, lower mass (allowing movement on smaller branches), and the ability to move through more cluttered habitat. Size relating to weight affects gliding animals such as the reduced weight per snout-vent length for 'flying' frogs.

Hanging Under Perches: Some species of primate, bats, and all species of sloth achieve passive stability by hanging beneath the branch. Both pitching and tipping become irrelevant, as the only method of failure would be losing their grip.

Behavioural Specialisations: Arboreal species have behaviours specialised for moving in their habitats, most prominently in terms of posture and gait. Specifically, arboreal mammals take longer steps, extend their limbs further forwards and backwards during a step, adopt a more 'crouched' posture to lower their centre of mass, and use a diagonal sequence gait.

Ecological consequences: Arboreal locomotion allows animals access to different resources, depending upon their abilities. Larger species may be restricted to larger-diametre branches that can support their weight, while smaller species may avoid competition by moving in the narrower branches.

Climbing Without Trees: Many animals climb in other habitats, such as in rock piles or mountains, and in those habitats, many of the same principles apply due to inclines, narrow ledges, and balance issues. However, less research has been conducted on the specific demands of locomotion in these habitats.

Perhaps the most exceptional of the animals that move on steep or even near vertical rock faces by careful balancing and leaping are the various types of mountain dwelling caprid such as the Barbary sheep, markhor, yak, ibex, tahr, rocky mountain goat, and chamois. Their adaptations may include a soft rubbery pad between their hooves for grip, hooves with sharp keratin rims for lodging in small footholds, and prominent dew claws. The snow leopard, being a predator of such mountain caprids, also has spectacular balance and leaping abilities; being able to leap up to ~17m (~50 ft). Other balancers and leapers include the mountain zebra, mountain tapir, and hyraxes.

Brachiation

Brachiation is a specialised form of arboreal locomotion, used by primates to move very rapidly while hanging beneath branches. Arguably the epitome of arboreal locomotion, it involves swinging with the arms from one handhold to another.

Only a few species are brachiators, and all of these are primates; it is a major means of locomotion among spider monkeys and gibbons, and is occasionally used by female orangutans. Gibbons are the experts of this mode of locomotion, swinging from branch to branch distances of up to 15 m (50 ft), and traveling at speeds of as much as 56 km/h (35 mph).

Gliding between Trees: To bridge gaps between trees, many animals such as the flying squirrel have adapted membranes, such as patagia for gliding flight.

Limbless Climbing: Many species of snake are highly arboreal, and some have evolved specialised musculature for this habitat. While moving in arboreal habitats, snakes move slowly along bare branches using a specialised form of concertina locomotion, but when secondary branches emerge from the branch being moved on, snakes use lateral undulation, a much faster mode. As a result, snakes perform best on small perches in cluttered environments, while limbed organisms seem to do best on large perches in uncluttered environments.

Arboreal Animals

Many species of animals are arboreal, far too many to list individually. This list is of prominently or predominantly arboreal species and higher taxa.

- Primates
- Cats
- brushtail possums
- opossums
- Sloths
- Anteaters
- Treeshrews
- Goats
- Colugos
- Kinkajous
- Viverrids
- Many rodents
- Parrots
- Geckos
- Chameleons
- Many other lizards
- Mambas
- Brown Tree Snakes
- Many other snakes
- Stick insects
- Many other arthropods
- Tree snails
- Koalas.

Flying and Gliding Animals

A number of animals have evolved aerial locomotion, either by powered flight or by gliding. Flying and gliding animals have evolved separately many times, without any single ancestor. Flight has evolved at least four times, in the insects, pterosaurs, birds, and bats.

Gliding has evolved on many more occasions. Usually the development is to aid canopy animals in getting from tree to tree, although there are other possibilities. Gliding, in particular, has evolved among rainforest animals, especially in the rainforests in Asia (most especially Borneo) where the trees are tall and widely spaced. Several species of aquatic animals, and a few amphibious animals have also evolved to acquire this gliding flight ability, typically as a means of evading predators.

Types of Aerial Locomotion

- *Falling:* decreasing altitude under the force of gravity, using no adaptations to increase drag or provide lift.
- *Parachuting:* falling at an angle greater than 45° from the horizontal with adaptations to increase drag forces. Very small animals may be carried up by the wind. Some gliding animals may use their gliding membranes for drag rather than lift, to safely descend.
- *Gliding flight:* falling at an angle less than 45° from the horizontal with lift from adapted aerofoil membranes. This allows slowly falling directed horizontal movement, with streamlining to decrease drag forces for aerofoil efficiency and often with some maneuverability in air. Gliding animals have a lower aspect ratio (wing length/ breadth) than true flyers.
- *Flapping:* moving wings for directly producing thrust. May ascend without the aid of the wind, as opposed to gliders and parachuters.
- *Soaring:* gliding in rising or otherwise moving air that requires specific physiological and morphological adaptations that can sustain the animal aloft without flapping its wings. The rising air is due to thermals, ridge lift or other meteorological features. Under the right conditions, soaring creates a gain of altitude without expending energy. Large wingspans are needed for efficient soaring.
- *Ballooning:* being carried up into the air from the aerodynamic effect on long strands of silk in the wind. Certain silk-producing arthropods, mostly small or young spiders, secrete a special light-weight gossamer silk for ballooning, sometimes traveling great distances at high altitude.

These forms of aerial locomotion are not mutually exclusive and indeed many animals will employ two or more of the methods.

Two other common forms of aerial locomotion for humans that are not employed in the rest of the animal kingdom are heli-propulsion and lighter-than-air flight.

Ecology of Aerial Locomotion

Although only four groups of animals have evolved flight, all of the three extant groups are very successful, suggesting that flight is a very successful strategy once evolved. Bats, after rodents, have the most species of any mammalian order, about 20% of all mammalian species. Birds have the most species of any class of terrestrial vertebrates. Finally insects have more species than all other animal groups combined.

Flying animals may have evolved from gliding animals. However, gliding is not necessarily just an evolutionary route to flying and has some advantages of its own. Gliding is a very energy-efficient way of travelling from tree to tree. An argument made is that many gliding animals eat low energy foods such as leaves and are restricted to gliding because of this, whereas flying animals eat more high energy foods such as fruits, nectar, and insects. In contrast to flight, gliding has evolved independently many times (more than a dozen times among extant vertebrates), however these groups have not radiated nearly as much as have groups of flying animals.

One point of interest is the distribution of gliding animals. Most gliding animals live in rain forests (although a few gliding squirrels live in northern Asian and North American forests). Many gliding animals are found in Southeast Asia and some in Africa, whereas only a very few gliding vertebrates are found in South America (a handful of hylid frogs), India, or New Guinea (and none in Madagascar) despite seemingly suitable rain forest habitat.

However, many more animals in South America have prehensile tails than in Africa and Southeast Asia. It has been argued that gliding animals dominate in Southeast Asia as the forests are less dense than in South America. In dense forest there is not room to glide, but a prehensile tail is very useful for moving from tree to tree. Also South American rainforests tend to have more lianas as there are fewer large animals to eat them compared to Africa and Asia; these lianas would aid climbers but obstruct gliders. Curiously, Australia contains many mammals with prehensile tails and also many mammals which can glide; in fact, all Australian mammalian gliders have tails that are prehensile to an extent. Other theories for the higher number of gliding animals in Southeast Asian forests include the fact that the dominant canopy trees in such forests (mostly dipterocarp family trees) are taller than the canopy trees in other forests (gliders can glide further, from higher starting points, and travel further in such forests, giving them a competitive advantage) and the lower abundance of insect and small vertebrate prey for carnivorous animals (such as lizards) in such Asian forests (gliding predators may search wide areas for prey and mates more efficiently). Only a few animals are known to have specialised in soaring: the larger of the extinct pterosaurs, and some large birds. Powered flight is very energetically expensive for large animals, but for soaring their size is an advantage, as it allows them a low wing loading, that is a large wing areas relative to their weight, which maximizes lift. Soaring is very energetically efficient.

Biomechanics of Aerial Locomotion

The forms of aerial locomotion for which the biomechanics are most studied are bird flight and insect flight. The UCMP exhibit on vertebrate flight contains a broad introduction to the biomechanics of flying and gliding vertebrates.

Limits and Extremes

Flying/soaring:

- Largest. The largest known flying animal was formerly thought to be *Pteranodon*, a pterosaur with a wingspan of up to 7.5 m. However, the more recently discovered azhdarchid pterosaur *Quetzalcoatlus* is much larger, with estimates of the wingspan ranging from 9 m to 12 m. Some other recently discovered azhdarchid pterosaur species, such as *Hatzegopteryx*, may have also wingspans of a similar size or even slightly larger. Although it is widely thought that Quetzalcoatlus reached the size limit of a flying animal, it should be noted that the same was once said of Pteranodon. The heaviest living flying animals are the kori bustard and the great bustard with males reaching 21 kg. The wandering albatross has the greatest wingspan of any living flying animal at 3.63 m (11 ft 11 in). Among living animals which fly over land, the Andean condor and the marabou stork have the largest wingspan at 3.2 m. Studies have shown that it is physically possible for flying animals to reach 18 m (60 ft) wingspans, but there is no firm evidence that any flying animal, not even the azhdarchid pterosaurs, got that large.

- Smallest. There is no real minimum size for getting airborne. Indeed, there are many bacteria floating in the atmosphere that constitute part of the aeroplankton. However, to move about under one's own power and not be overly affected by the wind requires a certain amount of size. The smallest flying vertebrates are the bee hummingbird and the bumblebee bat, both of which may weigh less than 2 g. They are thought to represent the lower size limit for endotherm flight.
- Fastest. The fastest of all known flying animals is the peregrine falcon, which when diving has been recorded flying at 300 km/h or faster. The fastest animal in flapping flight might be the White-throated Needle-tailed Swift, at 170 km/h. In level flapping flight, a good contender for the fastest living animal recorded is the red-breasted merganser at 160 km/h (100 mi/h).
- Slowest. Most flying animals need to travel forward at a minimum speed to stay aloft. However, some creatures can stay in the same spot, known as hovering, either by rapidly flapping the wings, as do hummingbirds, hoverflies, dragonflies, and some others, or carefully using thermals, as do some birds of prey. The slowest flying non-hovering bird recorded is the American woodcock, at 8 km/h. However, many insects probably fly much more slowly than this.
- Highest flying. There are records of a Rüppell's Vulture *Gyps rueppelli*, a large vulture, being sucked into a jet engine 11,550 m (37,900 feet) above Côte d'Ivoire in West Africa. The animal that flies highest most regularly is the bar-headed goose *Anser indicus*, which migrates directly over the Himalayas between its nesting grounds in Tibet and its winter quarters in India. They are

sometimes seen flying well above the peak of Mount Everest at 8,848 m (29,028 feet).

- Most maneuverable. A number of flying animals are known for their maneuverability. Many animals that can hover are often very maneuverable, being able to move in any direction as well as stay still. Other flying animals known for their aerial acrobatics are bats and crows.

Gliding/Parachuting

- Most efficient glider. This can be taken as the animal that moves most horizontal distance per metre fallen. Flying squirrels are known to glide up to 200 m, but have measured glide ratio of about 2. Flying fish have been observed to glide for hundreds of metres on the drafts on the edge of waves with only their initial leap from the water to provide height, but may be obtaining additional lift from wave motion. On the other hand Albatrosses have measured lift/drag ratios of 20, and thus fall just 1 metre for every 20 in still air.
- Most maneuverable glider. Many gliding animals have some ability to turn, but which is the most maneuverable is difficult to assess. Even Paradise tree snakes, Chinese gliding frogs, and gliding ants have been observed as having considerable capacity to turn in the air.

Animals Which Parachute, Glide, or Fly (Living)

Vertebrates

Fish:

- Flying fish (gliding). There are over 50 species of flying fish belonging to the family Exocoetidae. They are mostly marine fishes of small to medium size. The largest flying fish can reach lengths of 45 cm, but most species measure less than 30 cm in length. They can be divided into two-winged varieties and four-winged varieties. Before the fish leaves the water it increases its speed to around 30 body lengths per second and as it breaks the surface and is freed from the drag of the water it can be traveling at around 60 km/h. The glides are usually up to 30–50 metres in length, but some have been observed soaring for hundreds of metres using the updraft on the leading edges of waves. The fish can also make a series of glides, each time dipping the tail into the water to produce forward thrust. The longest recorded series of glides, with the fish only periodically dipping its tail in the water, was for 45 seconds (Video here). It has been suggested that the genus *Exocoetus* is on an evolutionary borderline between flight and gliding. It flaps its enlarged pectoral fins when airborne, but still seems only to glide, as there is no hint of a power stroke. It has been found that some flying fish can glide as effectively as some flying birds.

- Halfbeaks (gliding). A group related to the Exocoetidae, one or two hemirhamphid species possess enlarged pectoral fins and show true gliding flight rather than simple leaps. Marshall (1965) reports that *Euleptorhamphus viridis* can cover 50 m in two separate hops.
- Freshwater butterflyfish (possibly gliding). *Pantodon buchholzi* has the ability to jump and possibly glide a short distance. It can move through the air several times the length of its body. While it does this, the fish flaps its large pectoral fins, giving it its common name. However, it is debated whether the freshwater butterfly fish can truly glide, Saidel et al. (2004) argue that it cannot.
- Freshwater hatchetfish (possibly flying). There are 9 species of freshwater hatchetfish split among 3 genera. Freshwater hatchetfish have an extremely large sternal region that is fitted with a large amount of muscle that allows it to flap its pectoral fins. They can move in a straight line over a few metres to escape predators.

Amphibians:

- Rhacophoridae flying frogs (gliding). Gliding has evolved independently in two families of tree frogs, the Old World Rhacophoridae and the New World Hylidae. Within each lineage there are a range of gliding abilities from non-gliding, to parachuting, to full gliding. A number of the Rhacophoridae, such as Wallace's Flying Frog (*Rhacophorus nigropalmatus*), have adaptation for gliding, the main feature being enlarged toe membranes. For example, the Malayan flying frog glides using the membranes between the toes of its limbs, and small membranes located at the heel, the base of the leg, and the forearm. Some of the frogs are quite accomplished gliders, for example, the Chinese gliding frog *Polypedates dennysi* can maneuver in the air, making two kinds of turn, either rolling into the turn (a banked turn) or yawing into the turn (a crabbed turn).

- Hylidae flying frogs (gliding). The other frog family that contains gliders.

Reptiles:

- *Draco* lizards (gliding). There are 28 species of lizard of the genus *Draco,* found in Sri Lanka, India, and Southeast Asia. They live in trees, feeding on tree ants, but nest on the forest floor. They can glide for up to 60 m and over this distance they lose only 10 m in height. Unusually, their patagium (gliding membrane) is supported on elongated ribs rather than the more common situation among gliding vertebrates of having the patagium attached to the limbs. When extended, the ribs form a semicircle on either side the lizard's body and can be folded to the body like a folding fan.
- Gliding Lacertids (gliding). There are two species of gliding lacertid, of the genus *Holaspis.* Found in Africa. They have fringed toes and tail sides and can flatten their bodies for gliding/parachuting.
- *Ptychozoon* flying geckos (gliding). There are six species of gliding gecko, of the genus *Ptychozoon,* from Southeast Asia. These lizards have small flaps of skin along their limbs, torso, tail, and head that catch the air and enable them to glide.
- *Lupersaurus* flying geckos (gliding). A possible sister-taxon to Ptychozoon which has similar flaps and folds and also glides.
- *Thecadactylus* flying geckos (gliding). At least some species of Thecadactylus, such as T. rapicauda, are known to glide.
- *Cosymbotus* flying gecko (gliding). Similar adaptations to Ptychozoon are found in the two species of the gecko genus *Cosymbotus.*

- *Chrysopelea* snakes (gliding). Five species of snake from Southeast Asia, Melanesia, and India. The paradise tree snake of southern Thailand, Malaysia, Borneo, Philippines, and Sulawesi is the most capable glider of those snakes studied. It glides by stretching out its body sideways and opening its ribs so the belly is concave, and by making lateral slithering movements. It can remarkably glide up to 100 m and make 90 degree turns.

Birds:

- Birds (flying, soaring) - Most of the approximately 10,000 living species can fly, (flightless birds are the exception). Bird flight is one of the most studied forms of aerial locomotion in animals.

Mammals:

- Flying phalangers or wrist-winged gliders (subfamily Petaurinae) (gliding). Possums found in Australia, and New Guinea. The gliding membranes are hardly noticeable until they jump. On jumping, the animal extends all four legs and stretches the loose but muscularly controlled folds of skin. The subfamily contains seven species. Of the six species in the genus Petaurus, the Sugar glider and the Biak Glider are the most common species. The lone species in the genus Gymnobelideus, Leadbeater's Possum has only a vestigial gliding membrane.
- Greater glider (*Petauroides volans*) (gliding). The only species of the genus Petauroidae of the family Pseudocheiridae. This Marsupial is found in Australia, and was originally classed with the flying phalangers, but is now recognised as separate. Its flying membrane only extends to the elbow, rather than to the wrist as in Petaurinae.
- Feather-tailed possums (family Acrobatidae) (gliding). This family of Marsupials contains two genera, each with one species. The Feathertail Glider (*Acrobates pygmaeus*), found in Australia is the size of a very small mouse and is the smallest mammalian glider. The Feathertail Possum (*Distoechurus pennatus*) is found in New Guinea, but does not glide. Both species have a stiff-haired feather-like tail.

- Bats (flying). There are approximately 1,240 bat species, representing about 20% of all classified mammal species.
- Flying squirrels (subfamily Petauristinae) (gliding). There are 43 species divided between 14 genera of flying squirrel. Flying squirrels are found almost worldwide in tropical (Southeast Asia, India, and Sri Lanka), temperate, and even Arctic environments. They tend to be nocturnal. When a flying squirrel wishes to cross to a tree that is further away than the distance possible by jumping, it extends the cartilage spur on its elbow or wrist. This opens out the flap of furry skin (the patagium) that stretches from its wrist to its ankle. It glides spread-eagle and with its tail fluffed out like a parachute, and grips the tree with its claws when it lands. Flying squirrels have been reported to glide over 200 m.
- Anomalure or scaly-tailed flying squirrels (Anomaluridae family) (gliding). These brightly coloured African rodents are not squirrels but have evolved to a resemble flying squirrels by convergent evolution. There are seven species, divided in three genera. All but one species have gliding membranes between their front and hind legs. The genus *Idiurus* contains two particularly small species known as flying mice, but similarly they are not true mice.
- Colugos or Flying lemurs (order Dermoptera) (gliding). There are two species of flying lemur. This is not a lemur, which is a primate, but molecular evidence suggests that colugos are a sister group to primates; however, some mammologists suggest they are a sister group to bats. Found in Southeast Asia, the colugo is probably the mammal most adapted for gliding, with a patagium that is as large as geometrically possible. They can glide as far as 70 m with minimal loss of height.
- Sifaka and possibly some other primates (possible limited gliding/parachuting). A number of primates have been suggested to have adaptations that allow limited gliding and/or parachuting: sifakas, indris, galagos and saki monkeys. Most notably, the sifaka, a type of lemur,

has thick hairs on its forearms that have been argued to provide drag, and a small membrane under its arms that has been suggested to provide lift by having aerofoil properties.

- Cats and maybe others. (very limited parachuting). If they fall cats spread their bodies to maximize drag, a very limited form of parachuting. Cats have an innate 'righting reflex' that allows them to rotate their bodies so they fall feet first. Some other animals may show similar very limited parachuting. There are also anecdotal accounts of less limited parachuting, or even semi-gliding, in palm civets.

Animals Which Parachute, Glide, or fly (Extinct)

Reptiles:

- Extinct reptiles similar to *Draco* (gliding). There are a number of unrelated extinct lizard-like reptiles with similar "wings" to the *Draco* lizards. *Icarosaurus, Daedalosaurus, Coelurosauravus, Weigeltosaurus, Mecistotrachelos*, and *Kuehneosaurus*. The largest of these, *Kuehneosaurus*, has a wingspan of 30 cm, and was estimated to be able to glide about 30 m.
- *Sharovipteryx* (gliding). This strange reptile, sometimes proposed as a pterosaur ancestor, from the Upper Triassic of Kirghiia unusually had a membrane on its elongated hind limbs, as opposed to the forelimbs, which is much more usual. In some reconstructions they had webbing on the forelimbs and neck as well.
- *Longisquama insignis* (possibly gliding/parachuting). This small reptile may have had long paired feather-like scales on its back, however it has been more recently argued that the scales form just a single dorsal frill. If paired, they may have been used for parachuting. "Everything you can make out is consistent with it being a small, tree-living, gliding animal, which is precisely the thing you'd expect birds to evolve out of," says Larry Martin, senior curator at the Natural History Museum at the University of Kansas.
- Pterosaurs (flying). Pterosaurs were the first flying vertebrates, and are generally agreed to have been

sophisticated flyers. They had large wings formed by a patagium stretching from the torso to a dramatically lengthened fourth finger. There were hundreds of species, most of which are thought to have been intermittent flappers, and many soarers. The largest known flying animals are pterosaurs.

Birds:

- Theropods (gliding/flying). There were several species of theropod dinosaur thought to be capable of gliding or flying, that are not classified as birds (though they are closely related). Some species (*Microraptor gui*, *Microraptor zhaoianus*, and *Cryptovolans pauli*) have been found that were fully feathered on all four limbs, giving them four 'wings' that they are believed to have used for gliding or flying.

Mammals:

- *Volaticotherium antiquum* (gliding). The earliest known flying or gliding mammal. This squirrel-sized animal belonged to a now extinct ancestral line and was not related to modern day flying or gliding mammals, such as bats or gliding marsupials. It lived at least 125 million years ago and used a fur-covered skin membrane to glide through the air.
- Several species of extinct bat have been found, like *Icaronycteris*, *Palaeochiropteryx*, and *Onychonycteris*.

Feeding

To maintain a high constant body temperature is energy expensive – mammals therefore need a nutritious and plentiful diet. While the earliest mammals were probably predators, different species have since adapted to meet their dietary requirements in a variety of ways. Some eat other animals – this is a carnivorous diet (and includes insectivorous diets). Other mammals, called herbivores, eat plants. A herbivorous diet includes subtypes such as fruit-eating and grass-eating. An omnivore eats both prey and plants.

Carnivorous mammals have a simple digestive tract, because the proteins, lipids, and minerals found in meat require little in the way of specialised digestion. Plants, on the other hand, contain complex carbohydrates, such as cellulose. The digestive tract of an herbivore is therefore host to bacteria that ferment these substances, and make them available for digestion. The bacteria are either housed in the multichambered stomach or in a large cecum.

The size of an animal is also a factor in determining diet type. Since small mammals have a high ratio of heat-losing surface area to heat-generating volume, they tend to have high energy requirements and a high metabolic rate. Mammals that weigh less than about 18 oz (500 g) are mostly insectivorous because they cannot tolerate the slow, complex digestive process of a herbivore. Larger animals, on the other hand, generate more heat and less of this heat is lost.

They can therefore tolerate either a slower collection process (those that prey on larger vertebrates) or a slower digestive process (herbivores). Furthermore, mammals that weigh more than 18 oz (500 g) usually cannot collect enough insects during their waking hours to sustain themselves. The only large insectivorous mammals are those that feed on huge colonies of insects (ants or termites). Specialisations in herbivory include: Granivory "seed eating", folivory "leaf eating", frugivory "fruit eating", nectivory "nectar eating", gumivory "gum eating", and mycophagy "fungus eating".

Chapter 2

Integumentary System

The integumentary system is the organ system that protects the body from damage, comprising the skin and its appendages (including hair, scales, feathers, hoofs, and nails). The integumentary system has a variety of functions; it may serve to waterproof, cushion, and protect the deeper tissues, excrete wastes, and regulate temperature, and is the attachment site for sensory receptors to detect pain, sensation, pressure, and temperature. In most terrestrial vertebrates with significant exposure to sunlight, the integumentary system also provides for vitamin D synthesis.

Layers of the Skin

The integumentary system is the largest of the body's organ systems. In humans, this system accounts for about 12 to 15 percent of total body weight and covers 1.5-2m^2 of surface area. It distinguishes, separates, and protects the organism from its surroundings. Small-bodied invertebrates of aquatic or continually moist habitats respire using the outer layer (integument). This gas exchange system, where gases simply diffuse into and out of the interstitial fluid, is called integumentary exchange.

The human skin (integument) is composed of a minimum of 3 major layers of tissue: the epidermis; dermis; and hypodermis. The epidermis forms the outermost layer, providing the initial barrier to the external environment. Beneath this, the dermis comprises two sections, the papillary and reticular layers, and contains connective tissues, vessels, glands, follicles, hair roots, sensory nerve endings, and muscular tissue. The deepest layer is the hypodermis, which is primarily made up of adipose tissue. Substantial collagen bundles anchor the dermis to the hypodermis in a way that permits most areas of the skin to move freely over the deeper tissue layers.

Epidermis (Skin)

The epidermis is composed of the outermost layers of cells in the skin, "epi" in Greek meaning "over" or "upon", which together with the dermis forms the cutis. The epidermis is a stratified squamous epithelium, composed of proliferating basal and differentiated suprabasal keratinocytes which acts as the body's major barrier against an inhospitable environment, by preventing pathogens from entering, making the skin a natural barrier to infection. It also regulates the amount of water released from the body into the atmosphere through transepidermal water loss (TEWL). In humans, it is thinnest on the eyelids at 0.05 mm (0.0020 in) and thickest on the palms and soles at 1.5 mm (0.059 in). It is ectodermal in origin.

Structure

Cellular Components: The epidermus is avascular, nourished by diffusion from the dermis, constituted at 95% of keratinocytes but also containing melanocytes, Langerhans cells, Merkel cells, and inflammatory cells. *Rete ridges* ("rete tips") are epidermal thickenings that extend downward between dermal papillae. Blood capillaries are found beneath the epidermis, and are linked to an arteriole and a venule. Arterial shunt vessels may bypass the network in ears, the nose and fingertips.

Layers

The epidermis is composed of 4 or 5 layers depending on the region of skin being considered. Those layers in descending order are:

- cornified layer (*stratum corneum*)

Composed of 10 to 30 layers of polyhedral, anucleated corneocytes (final step of keratinocyte differentiation), with the palms and soles having the most layers.

- clear/translucent layer (*stratum lucidum*, only in palms and soles)

- granular layer (*stratum granulosum*)

Keratinocytes lose their nuclei and their cytoplasm appears granular. Lipids, contained into those keratinocytes within lamellar bodies, are released into the extracellular space through exocytosis to form a lipid barrier. Those polar lipids are then converted into non-polar lipids and arranged parallel to the cell surface. For example glycosphingolipids become ceramides and phospholipids become free fatty acids.

- spinous layer (*stratum spinosum*)

Keratinocytes become connected through desmosomes and start produce lamellar bodies, from within the Golgi, enriched in polar lipids, glycosphingolipids, free sterols, phospholipids and catabolic enzymes. Langerhans cells, immunologically active cells, are located in the middle of this layer.

- basal/germinal layer (*stratum basale/germinativum*).

Composed mainly of proliferating and non-proliferating keratinocytes, attached to the basement membrane by hemidesmosomes. Melanocytes are present, connected to numerous keratinocytes in this and other strata through dendrites.

Merkel cells are also found in the stratum basale with large numbers in touch-sensitive sites such as the fingertips and lips. They are closely associated with cutaneous nerves and seem to be involved in light touch sensation. The term Malpighian layer (*stratum malpighi*) is usually defined as both the stratum basale and stratum spinosum. The epidermis is separated from the dermis, its underlying tissue, by a basement membrane.

Cellular Kinyotics

Cell Division: The stratified squamous epithelium is maintained by cell division within the stratum basale. Differentiating cell delaminate from the basement membrane and are displaced outwards through the epidermal layers, undergoing multiple stages of differentiation until, in the stratum corneum, losing their nucleus and fusing to squamous sheets, which are eventually shed from the surface (desquamation). Differentiated keratinocytes secrete keratin proteins which contribute to the formation of an extracellular matrix and is an integral part of the skin barrier function. In normal skin, the rate of keratinocyte production equals the rate of loss, taking about two weeks for a cell to journey from the stratum basale to the top of the stratum granulosum, and an additional four weeks to cross the stratum corneum. The entire epidermis is replaced by new cell growth over a period of about 48 days.

Calcium Concentration

Keratinocyte differentiation throughout the epidermis is in part mediated by a calcium gradient, increasing from the stratum basale until the outer stratum granulosum, where it reaches its maximum, and decreasing in the stratum corneum. Calcium concentration in the stratum corneum is very low in part because those relatively dry cells are not able to dissolve the ions. This calcium gradient parallels keratinocyte differentiation and as such is considered a key regulator in the formation of the epidermal layers.

Elevation of extracellular calcium concentrations induces an increase in intracellular free calcium concentrations. Part of that intracellular increase comes from calcium released from intracellular stores and another part comes from transmembrane calcium influx, through both calcium-sensitive chloride channels and voltage-independent cation channels permeable to calcium. Moreover, it has been suggested that an extracellular calcium-sensing receptor (CaSR) also contributes to the rise in intracellular calcium concentration.

Organogenesis

Epidermal organogenesis, the formation of the epidermis, begins in the cells covering the embryo after neurulation, the formation of the central nervous system. In most vertebrates, this original one-layered structure quickly transforms into a two-layered tissue; a temporary outer layer, the periderm, which is disposed once the inner basal layer or *stratum germinativum* has formed.

This inner layer is a germinal epithelium that give rise to all epidermal cells. It divides to form the outer spinous layer (*stratum spinosum*). The cells of these two layers, together called the Malpighian layer(s) after Marcello Malpighi, divide to form the superficial granular layer (*Stratum granulosum*) of the epidermis.

The cells in the stratum granulosum do not divide, but instead form skin cells called keratinocytes from the granules of keratin. These skin cells finally become the cornified layer (*stratum corneum*), the outermost epidermal layer, where the cells become flattened sacks with their nuclei located at one end of the cell. After birth these outermost cells are replaced by new cells from the stratum granulosum and throughout life they are shed at a rate of 1.5 g (0.053 oz) per day.

Epidermal development is a product of several growth factors, two of which are:

- Transforming growth factor Alpha (TGFá) is an autocrine growth factor by which basal cells stimulate their own division.
- Keratinocyte growth factor (KGF or FGF7) is a paracrine growth factor produced by the underlying dermal fibroblasts in which the proliferation of basal cells is regulated.

Function

Barrier: The epidermis serves as a barrier to protect the body against microbial pathogens, oxidant stress (UV light) and chemical compounds and provides mechanical resistance. Most of that function is played by the stratum corneum.

Characteristics of the Barrier

- Physical barrier through keratinocytes attached together via cell–cell junctions and associated to cytoskeletal proteins, which gives the epidermis its mechanical strength.
- Chemical barrier through the presence of highly organised lipids, acids, hydrolytic enzymes and antimicrobial peptides.
- Immunologically active barrier through humoral and cellular constituents of the immune system.
- Water content of the stratum corneum drops towards the surface, creating hostile conditions for pathogenic microorganism growth.

- An acidic pH (around 5.0) and low amounts of water make it hostile to many microorganic pathogens.
- The presence of non-pathogenic microorganism on the epidermis surface help defend against pathogenic one by limiting food availability and through chemical secretions.

Factors That will Alter the Barrier

- Psychological stress, through an increase in glucocorticoids, compromises the stratum corneum and thus the barrier function.
- Sudden and large shifts in humidity alter stratum corneum hydration in a way that could allow entry of pathogenic microorganisms.

Skin Hydration

The ability of the skin to hold water is primarily due to the stratum corneum and is critical for maintaining healthy skin. Lipids arranged through a gradient and in an organised manner between the cells of the stratum corneum form a barrier to transepidermal water loss.

Skin Colour

The amount and distribution of melanin pigment in the epidermis is the main reason for variation in skin colour in Homo sapiens. Melanin is found in the small melanosomes, particles formed in melanocytes from where they are transferred to the surrounding keratinocytes. The size, number, and arrangement of the melanosomes varies between racial groups, but while the number of melanocytes can vary between different body regions, their numbers remain the same in individual body regions in all human beings. In white and oriental skin the melanosomes are packed in "aggregates", but in black skin they are larger and distributed more evenly. The number of melanosomes in the keratinocytes increases with UV radiation exposure, while their distribution remain largely unaffected.

Culture: Laboratory culture of keratinocytes to form a 3D structure (artificial skin) recapitulating most of the properties of the epidermis is routinely used as a tool for drug development and testing.

Dermis

The dermis is a layer of skin between the epidermis (with which it makes up the cutis) and subcutaneous tissues, that consists of connective tissue and cushions the body from stress and strain. It is divided into two layers, the superficial area adjacent to the epidermis called the papillary region and a deep thicker area known as the reticular dermis.

The dermis is tightly connected to the epidermis through a basement membrane. Structural components of the dermis are collagen, elastic fibres, and extrafibrillar matrix (previously called ground substance).

It also contains Mechanoreceptors that provide the sense of touch and heat, hair follicles, sweat glands, sebaceous glands, apocrine glands, lymphatic vessels and blood vessels. Those blood vessels provide nourishment and waste removal for both dermal and epidermal cells.

Components of the Dermis

The dermis is composed of three major types of cells: Fibroblasts, Macrophages, and Adipocytes. Apart from these cells, the dermis is also composed of matrix components such as collagen (which provides strength), elastin (which provides elasticity), the epidermis, and glycosaminoglycans.

Layers

Stratum Papillare: The papillary region is composed of loose areolar connective tissue. This is named for its fingerlike projections called *papillae*, that extend toward the epidermis and contain either terminal networks of blood capillaries or tactile Meissner's corpuscles.

Stratum Reticulare: The reticular region lies under the papillary region and is usually much thicker. It is composed of dense irregular connective tissue, and receives its name from the dense concentration of collagenous, elastic, and reticular fibres that weave throughout it.

These protein fibres give the dermis its properties of strength, extensibility, and elasticity. Also located within the reticular region are the roots of the hair, sebaceous glands, sweat glands, receptors, nails, and blood vessels.

Embryology

Embryology (from Greek —ìâñõïí, *embryon*, "the unborn, embryo"; and -ëïãßá, *-logia*) is the science of the development of an embryo from the fertilization of the ovum to the fetus stage.

Embryonic Development of Animals: After cleavage, the dividing cells, or morula, becomes a hollow ball, or blastula, which develops a hole or pore at one end.

Bilaterans

In bilateral animals, the blastula develops in one of two ways that divides the whole animal kingdom into two halves. If in the blastula the first pore (blastopore) becomes the mouth of the animal, it is a protostome; if the first pore becomes the anus then it is a deuterostome.

The protostomes include most invertebrate animals, such as insects, worms and molluscs, while the deuterostomes include the vertebrates. In due course, the blastula changes into a more differentiated structure called the gastrula.

The Gastrula with its Blastopore Soon Develops three Distinct Layers of Cells (the Germ Layers) from Which all the Bodily Organs and Tissues then Develop:

- The innermost layer, or endoderm, gives rise to the digestive organs, the gills, lungs or swim bladder if present, and kidneys or nephrites.
- The middle layer, or mesoderm, gives rise to the muscles, skeleton if any, and blood system.
- The outer layer of cells, or ectoderm, gives rise to the nervous system, including the brain, and skin or carapace and hair, bristles, or scales.

Embryos in many species often appear similar to one another in early developmental stages.

The reason for this similarity is because species have a shared evolutionary history.

These similarities among species are called homologous structures, which are structures that have the same or similar function and mechanism, having evolved from a common ancestor.

Humans

Humans are bilaterans and deuterostomes—the anus develops first. In humans, the term embryo refers to the ball of dividing cells from the moment the zygote implants itself in the uterus wall until the end of the eighth week after conception. Beyond the eighth week after conception (tenth week of pregnancy), the developing human is then called a fetus.

History of Embryology

As recently as the 18th century, the prevailing notion in human embryology was preformation: the idea that semen contains an embryo — a preformed, miniature infant, or "*homunculus*" — that simply becomes larger during development. The competing explanation of embryonic development was *epigenesis*, originally proposed 2,000 years earlier by Aristotle. Much early embryology came from the work of the great Italian anatomists: Aldrovandi, Aranzio, Leonardo da Vinci, Marcello Malpighi, Gabriele Falloppio, Girolamo Cardano, Emilio Parisano, Fortunio Liceti, Stefano Lorenzini, Spallanzani, Enrico Sertoli, Mauro Rusconi, etc. According to epigenesis, the form of an animal emerges gradually from a relatively formless egg. As microscopy improved during the 19th century, biologists could see that embryos took shape in a series of progressive steps, and epigenesis displaced preformation as the favoured explanation among embryologists.

After 1827

Karl Ernst von Baer and Heinz Christian Pander proposed the germ layer theory of development; von Baer discovered the mammalian ovum in 1827. Modern embryological pioneers include Charles Darwin, Ernst Haeckel, J.B.S. Haldane, and Joseph Needham. Other important contributors include William Harvey, Kaspar Friedrich Wolff, Heinz Christian Pander, August Weismann, Gavin de Beer, Ernest Everett Just, and Edward B. Lewis.

After 1950

After the 1950s, with the DNA helical structure being unravelled and the increasing knowledge in the field of molecular biology, developmental biology emerged as a field of study which attempts to correlate the genes with morphological change, and so tries to determine which genes are responsible for each morphological change that takes place in an embryo, and how these genes are regulated.

Vertebrate and Invertebrate Embryology

Many principles of embryology apply to invertebrates as well as to vertebrates. Therefore, the study of invertebrate embryology has advanced the study of vertebrate embryology. However, there are many differences as well. For example, numerous invertebrate species release a larva before development is complete; at the end of the larval period, an animal for the first time comes to resemble an adult similar to its parent or parents.

Although invertebrate embryology is similar in some ways for different invertebrate animals, there are also countless variations. For instance, while spiders proceed directly from egg to adult form many insects develop through at least one larval stage

Human Vertebral Column

In human anatomy, the vertebral column (Latin " *Columna vertebralis*) (backbone or spine) is a column usually consisting of 24 articulating vertebrae, and 9 fused vertebrae in the sacrum and the coccyx.

It is situated in the dorsal aspect of the torso, separated by intervertebral discs. It houses and protects the spinal cord in its spinal canal.

There are normally thirty-three (33) vertebrae in humans, including the five that are fused to form the sacrum (the others are separated by intervertebral discs) and the four coccygeal bones that form the *tailbone*.

The upper three regions comprise the remaining 24, and are grouped under the names *cervical* (7 vertebrae), *thoracic* (12 vertebrae) and *lumbar* (5 vertebrae), according to the regions they occupy.

This number is sometimes increased by an additional vertebra in one region, or it may be diminished in one region, the deficiency often being supplied by an additional vertebra in another. The number of cervical vertebrae is, however, very rarely increased or diminished.

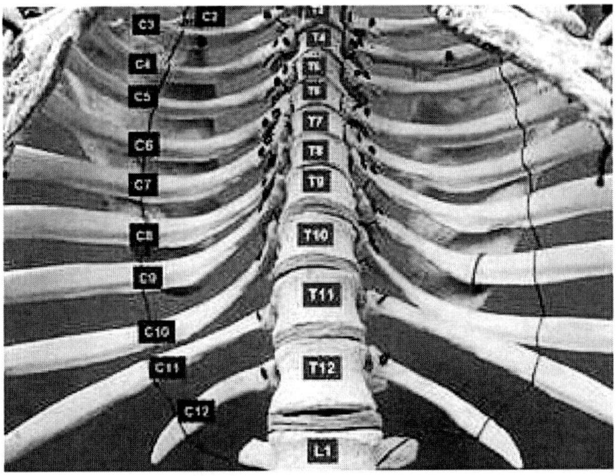

Figure: *Vertebral column*

With the exception of the first and second cervical, the true or movable vertebrae (the upper three regions) present certain common characteristics that are best studied by examining one from the middle of the thoracic region.

Structure of Individual Vertebrae

When the vertebrae are articulated with each other, the bodies form a strong pillar for the support of the head and trunk, and the vertebral foramina constitute a canal for the protection of the *medulla spinalis* (spinal cord). In between every pair of vertebrae are two apertures, the intervertebral foramina, one on either side, for the transmission of the spinal nerves and vessels. Two transverse processes and one spinous process are posterior to (behind) the vertebral body. The spinous process comes out the back, one transverse process comes out the left, and one on the right. The spinous processes of the cervical and lumbar regions can be felt through the skin. Superior and inferior articular facets on each vertebra act to restrict the range of movement possible. These facets are joined by a thin portion of the neural arch called the *pars interarticularis*.

Curves

Viewed laterally the vertebral column presents several curves, which correspond to the different regions of the column, and are called cervical, thoracic, lumbar, and pelvic. The cervical curve, convex forward, begins at the apex of the odontoid (*tooth-like*) process, and ends at the middle of the second thoracic vertebra; it is the least marked of all the curves. The thoracic curve, concave forward, begins at the middle of the second and ends at the middle of the twelfth thoracic vertebra. Its most prominent point behind corresponds to the spinous process of the seventh thoracic vertebra. This curve is known as a *tt curve.*

The lumbar curve is more marked in the female than in the male; it begins at the middle of the last thoracic vertebra, and ends at the sacrovertebral angle. It is convex anteriorly, the convexity of the lower three vertebrae being much greater than that of the upper two. This curve is described as a *lordotic curve.* The pelvic curve begins at the sacrovertebral articulation, and ends at the point of the coccyx; its concavity is directed downward and forward. The thoracic and pelvic curves are termed primary curves, because they alone are present during fetal life. The cervical and lumbar curves are *compensatory* or *secondary*, and are developed after birth, the former when the child is able to hold up its head (at three or four months) and to sit upright (at nine months), the latter at twelve or eighteen months, when the child begins to walk.

Regions

There are a total of 33 vertebrae in the vertebral column, if assuming 4 coccygeal vertebrae.

The individual vertebrae, named according to region and position, from superior to inferior, are:

- *Cervical:* 7 vertebrae (C1–C7)
- *Thoracic:* 12 vertebrae (T1–T12)
- *Lumbar:* 5 vertebrae (L1–L5)
- *Sacral:* 5 (fused) vertebrae (S1–S5)
- *Coccygeal:* 4 (3–5) (fused) vertebrae (Tailbone)

Cervical Vertebrae

In vertebrates, cervical vertebrae (singular: *vertebra*) are those vertebrae immediately inferior to the skull. Thoracic vertebrae in all mammalian species are defined as those vertebrae that also carry a pair of ribs, and lie caudal to the cervical vertebrae. Further caudally follow the lumbar vertebrae, which also belong to the trunk, but do not carry ribs. In reptiles, all trunk vertebrae carry ribs and are called dorsal vertebrae.

In many species, though not in mammals, the cervical vertebrae bear ribs. In many other groups, such as lizards and saurischian dinosaurs, the cervical ribs are large; in birds, they are small and completely fused to the vertebrae. The transverse processes of mammals are homologous to the cervical ribs of other amniotes. In humans, cervical vertebrae are the smallest of the true vertebrae, and can be readily distinguished from those of the thoracic or lumbar regions by the presence of a foramen (hole) in each transverse process, through which passes the vertebral artery. The remainder of this article focuses upon human anatomy.

General Characteristics (C3-C6)

By convention, the cervical vertebrae are numbered, with the first one (C1) located closest to the skull and higher numbered vertebrae (C2-C7) proceeding away from the skull and down the spine. The general characteristics of the third through sixth cervical vertebrae are described here. The first, second, and seventh vertebrae are extraordinary, and are detailed later.

- The body of these four vertebrae is small, and broader from side to side than from front to back.
    - The *anterior* and *posterior surfaces* are flattened and of equal depth; the former is placed on a lower level than the latter, and its inferior border is prolonged downward, so as to overlap the upper and forepart of the vertebra below.
    - The *upper surface* is concave transversely, and presents a projecting lip on either side.
    - the *lower surface* is concave from front to back, convex from side to side, and presents laterally shallow concavities which receive the corresponding projecting lips of the underlying vertebra.
- The pedicles are directed laterally and backward, and are attached to the body midway between its upper and lower borders, so that the superior vertebral notch is

as deep as the inferior, but it is, at the same time, narrower.

- The laminae are narrow, and thinner above than below; the vertebral foramen is large, and of a triangular form.
- The spinous process is short and bifid, the two divisions being often of unequal size.
- The superior and inferior articular processes of cervical vertebrae have fused on either or both sides to form articular pillars, columns of bone that project laterally from the junction of the pedicle and lamina.
- The articular facets are flat and of an oval form:
  - o the *superior* face backward, upward, and slightly medially.
  - o the *inferior* face forward, downward, and slightly laterally.
- The transverse processes are each pierced by the foramen transversarium, which, in the upper six vertebrae, gives passage to the vertebral artery and vein, as well as a plexus of sympathetic nerves. Each process consists of an anterior and a posterior part. These two parts are joined, outside the foramen, by a bar of bone that exhibits a deep sulcus on its upper surface for the passage of the corresponding spinal nerve.
  - o The anterior portion is the homologue of the rib in the thoracic region, and is therefore named the *costal process* or *costal element.* It arises from the side of the body, is directed laterally in front of the foramen, and ends in a tubercle, the anterior tubercle.
  - o The posterior part, the true transverse process, springs from the vertebral arch behind the foramen, and is directed forward and laterally; it ends in a flattened vertical tubercle, the posterior tubercle.

Special Cervical Vertebrae (C1, C2, and C7)

- *C1 or atlas:* The Atlas is the topmost vertebra, and – along with C2 – forms the joint connecting the skull and spine. Its chief peculiarity is that it has no body, and this is due to the fact that the body of the atlas has fused with that of the next vertebra.

- *C2 or axis:* It forms the pivot upon which C1 rotates. The most distinctive characteristic of this bone is the strong odontoid process (dens) that rises perpendicularly from the upper surface of the body. The body is deeper in front than behind, and prolonged downward anteriorly so as to overlap the upper and front part of the third vertebra.
- *C7 or vertebra prominens:* The most distinctive characteristic of this vertebra is the existence of a long and prominent spinous process, hence the name *vertebra prominens*. In some subjects, the seventh cervical vertebra is associated with an abnormal pair of ribs, known as cervical ribs. These ribs are usually small, but may occasionally compress blood vessels (such as the subclavian artery) or nerves in the brachial plexus, causing ischemic muscle pain, numbness, tingling, and weakness in the upper limb.

Movements of the Cervical Spine

The movement of nodding the head takes place predominantly through flexion and extension at the joint between the atlas and the occipital bone, the atlanto-occipital joint. However, the cervical spine is comparatively mobile, and some component of this movement is due to flexion and extension of the vertebral column itself.

The movement of shaking or rotating the head left and right happens almost entirely at the joint between the atlas and the axis, the atlanto-axial joint. A small amount of rotation of the vertebral column itself contributes to the movement.

Landmarks

Base of Nose and the Hard palate corresponds to C1.

Teeth (when mouth remains closed) correspond to C2.

Mandible and Hyoid bone correspond to C3.

The thyroid cartilage is from C4 to C5.

The cricoid cartilage is from C6 to C7.

Clinical Significance

Injuries to the cervical spine are common at the level of the second cervical vertebrae, but neurological injury is uncommon. If it does occur, however, it may cause death or profound disability, including paralysis of the arms, legs, and diaphragm, which leads to respiratory failure. Common patterns of injury include the odontoid fracture and the hangman's fracture, both of which are often treated with immobilization in a cervical collar or Halo brace.

A common EMS practice is to immobilize a patient's cervical spine to prevent further damage during transport to Medical Aid. This practice has come under review recently as incidence rates of unstable spinal trauma can be as low as 2% in immobilized patients. Canadian studies have developed the Canadian C-Spine Rule (CCR) for physicians to decide who should receive radiological imaging.

Thoracic Vertebrae

In vertebrates, thoracic vertebrae compose the middle segment of the vertebral column, between the cervical vertebrae and the lumbar vertebrae. In humans, they are intermediate in size between those of the cervical and lumbar regions; they increase in size as one proceeds down the spine, the upper vertebrae being much smaller than those in the lower part of the region.

They are distinguished by the presence of facets on the sides of the bodies for articulation with the heads of the ribs, and facets on the transverse processes of all, except the eleventh and twelfth, for articulation with the tubercles of the ribs.

Humans have 12, but numbers vary greatly; for example, most marsupials have 13, but koalas have only 11. 12 to 15 is common among mammals, with 18 to 20 in horses, tapirs, rhinoceroses, and elephants, and extremes in mammals are marked by certain sloths with 25 and cetaceans with 9. By convention, the human thoracic vertebrae are numbered, with the first one (T1) located closest to the skull and higher numbered vertebrae (T2-T12) proceeding away from the skull and down the spine.

General Characteristics

These are the general characteristics of the second through eighth thoracic vertebrae. The first and ninth through twelfth vertebrae contain certain peculiarities, and are detailed below.

The bodies in the middle of the thoracic region are heart-shaped, and as broad in the antero-posterior as in the transverse direction. At the ends of the thoracic region they resemble respectively those of the cervical and lumbar vertebrae. They are slightly thicker behind than in front, flat above and below, convex from side to side in front, deeply concave behind, and slightly constricted laterally and in front. They present, on either side, two costal demi-facets, one above, near the root of the pedicle, the other below, in front of the inferior vertebral notch; these are covered with cartilage in the fresh state, and, when the vertebrae are articulated with one another, form, with the intervening intervertebral fibrocartilages, oval surfaces for the reception of the heads of the ribs.

The pedicles are directed backward and slightly upward, and the inferior vertebral notches are of large size, and deeper than in any other region of the vertebral column. The laminae are broad, thick, and imbricated – that is to say, they overlap those of subjacent vertebrae like tiles on a roof. The vertebral foramen is small, and of a circular form. The spinous process is long, triangular on coronal section, directed obliquely downward, and ends in a tuberculated extremity. These processes overlap from the fifth to the eighth, but are less oblique in direction above and below.

The superior articular processes are thin plates of bone projecting upward from the junctions of the pedicles and laminae; their articular facets are practically flat, and are directed backward and a little lateralward and upward. The inferior articular processes are fused to a considerable extent with the laminae, and project but slightly beyond their lower borders; their facets are directed forward and a little medialward and downward.

The transverse processes arise from the arch behind the superior articular processes and pedicles; they are thick, strong, and of considerable length, directed obliquely backward and lateralward, and each ends in a clubbed extremity, on the front of which is a small, concave surface, for articulation with the tubercle of a rib.

Individual Thoracic Vertebrae

First Thoracic Vertebra: The first thoracic vertebra has, on either side of the body, an entire articular facet for the head of the first rib, and a demi-facet for the upper half of the head of the second rib. The body is like that of a cervical vertebra, being broad, concave, and lipped on either side.

The superior articular surfaces are directed upward and backward; the spinous process is thick, long, and almost horizontal.

The transverse processes are long, and the upper vertebral notches are deeper than those of the other thoracic vertebrae.

The thoracic spinal nerve 1 (T1) passes out underneath it.

Second Thoracic Vertebra: The thoracic spinal nerve 2 (T2) passes out underneath it. The second thoracic vertebra is larger than the first thoracic vertebra

Third Thoracic Vertebra: The thoracic spinal nerve 3 (T3) passes out underneath it.

Fourth Thoracic Vertebra: The fourth thoracic vertebra, together with the fifth, is at the same level as the sternal angle. The thoracic spinal nerve 4 (T4) passes out underneath it.

Fifth Thoracic Vertebra: The fifth thoracic vertebra, together with the fourth, is at the same level as the sternal angle. The human trachea divides into two main bronchi at the level of the 5th thoracic vertebra, but may also end higher or lower, depending on breathing. The thoracic spinal nerve 5 (T5) passes out underneath it.

Sixth Thoracic Vertebra: The thoracic spinal nerve 6 (T6) passes out underneath it.

Seventh Thoracic Vertebra: The thoracic spinal nerve 7 (T7) passes out underneath it.

Eighth Thoracic Vertebra: The eighth thoracic vertebra is, together with the ninth thoracic vertebra, at the same level as the xiphoid process. The thoracic spinal nerve 8 (T8) passes out underneath it.

Ninth Thoracic Vertebra: The ninth thoracic vertebra may have no demi-facets below. In some subjects however, it has two demi-facets on either side; when this occurs the tenth doesn't have facets but demi-facets at the upper part. The thoracic spinal nerve 9 (T9) passes out underneath it. The xiphisternum (or xiphoid process of the sternum) is at the same level in the axial plane.

Tenth Thoracic Vertebra: The tenth thoracic vertebra has (except in the cases just mentioned) an entire articular facet (not demi-facet) on either side, which is placed partly on the lateral surface of the pedicle. It doesn't have any kind of facet below, because the following ribs only have one facet on their heads. The thoracic spinal nerve 10 (T10) passes out underneath it.

Eleventh Thoracic Vertebra: In the eleventh thoracic vertebrae the body approaches in its form and size to that of the lumbar vertebrae.

The articular facets for the heads of the ribs are of large size, and placed chiefly on the pedicles, which are thicker and stronger in this and the next vertebrae than in any other part of the thoracic region.

The spinous process is short, and nearly horizontal in direction. The transverse processes are very short, tuberculated at their extremities, and do have articular facets. The thoracic spinal nerve 11 (T11) passes out underneath it.

Twelfth Thoracic Vertebra

The twelfth thoracic vertebra has the same general characteristics as the eleventh, but may be distinguished from it by its inferior articular surfaces being convex and directed lateralward, like those of the lumbar vertebrae; by the general form of the body, laminae, and spinous process, in which it resembles the lumbar vertebrae; and by each transverse process being subdivided into three elevations, the superior, inferior, and lateral tubercles: the superior and inferior correspond to the mammillary and accessory processes of the lumbar vertebrae. Traces of similar elevations are found on the transverse processes of the tenth and eleventh thoracic vertebrae. The thoracic spinal nerve 12 (T12) passes out underneath it.

Lumbar Vertebrae

In human anatomy, the lumbar vertebrae are the five vertebrae between the rib cage and the pelvis. They are the largest segments of the vertebral column and are characterized by the absence of the foramen transversarium within the transverse process, and by the absence of facets on the sides of the body. They are designated L1 to L5, starting at the top. The lumbar vertebrae help support the weight of the body, and permit movement.

Human Anatomy

General Characteristics: These are the general characteristics of the first through fourth lumbar vertebrae. The fifth vertebra contains certain peculiarities. As with other vertebrae, each lumbar vertebra consists of a *vertebral body* and a *vertebral arch*. The vertebral arch, consisting of a pair of *pedicles* and a pair of *laminae*, encloses the *vertebral foramen* (opening) and supports seven processes.

Body: The vertebral body of each lumbar vertebra is large, wider from side to side than from front to back, and a little thicker in front than in back. It is flattened or slightly concave above and below, concave behind, and deeply constricted in front and at the sides.

Arch: The pedicles are very strong, directed backward from the upper part of the vertebral body; consequently, the inferior vertebral notches are of considerable depth. The pedicles change in morphology from the upper lumbar to the lower lumbar. They increase in sagittal width from 9 mm to up to 18 mm at L5. They increase in angulation in the axial plane from 10 degrees to 20 degrees by L5. The pedicle is sometimes used as a portal of entrance into the vertebral body for fixation with pedicle screws or for placement of bone cement as with kyphoplasty or vertebroplasty. The laminae are broad, short, and strong. They form the posterior portion of the vertebral arch. In the upper lumbar region the lamina are taller than wide but in the lower lumbar vertebra the lamina are wider than tall. The lamina connect the spinous process to the pedicles. The vertebral foramen within the arch is triangular, larger than in the thoracic vertebrae, but smaller than in the cervical vertebrae.

Processes

The *spinous process* is thick, broad, and somewhat quadrilateral; it projects backward and ends in a rough, uneven border, thickest below where it is occasionally notched. The superior and inferior *articular processes* are well-defined, projecting respectively upward and downward from the junctions of pedicles and laminae. The facets on the superior processes are concave, and look backward and medialward; those on the inferior are convex, and are directed forward and lateralward. The former are wider apart than the latter, since in the articulated column the inferior articular processes are embraced by the superior processes of the subjacent vertebrate.

The *transverse processes* are long and slender. They are horizontal in the upper three lumbar vertebrae and incline a little upward in the lower two. In the upper three vertebrae they arise from the junctions of the pedicles and laminae, but in the lower two they are set farther forward and spring from the pedicles and posterior parts of the vertebral bodies.

They are situated in front of the articular processes instead of behind them as in the thoracic vertebrae, and are homologous with the ribs. Three portions or *tubercles* can be noticed in a transverse process of a lower lumbar vertebrae: the lateral or *costiform process*, the *mammillary process*, and the *accessory process*. The costiform is lateral, the mammillary is superior (cranial), and the accessory is inferior (caudal). The mammillary is connected in the lumbar region with the back part of the superior articular process. The accessory process is situated at the back part of the base of the transverse process. The tallest and thickest costiform process is usually that of L5.

First and Fifth Lumbar Vertebrae

The first lumbar vertebra is level with the anterior end of the ninth rib. This level is also called the important transpyloric plane, since the pylorus of the stomach is at this level. The fifth lumbar vertebra is characterized by its body being much deeper in front than behind, which accords with the prominence of the sacrovertebral articulation; by the smaller size of its spinous process; by the wide interval between the inferior articular processes, and by the thickness of its transverse processes, which spring from the body as well as from the pedicles. The fifth lumbar vertebra is by far the most common site of spondylolysis and spondylolisthesis. Most individuals have five lumbar vertebrae, while some have four or six. Lumbar disorders that normally affect L5 will affect L4 or L6 in these latter individuals.

Segmental Movements

The range of segmental movements in a single segment is difficult to measure clinically, not only because of variations between individuals, but also because it is age and gender dependent. Furthermore, flexion and extension in the lumbal spine is the product of a combination of rotation and translation in the sagittal plane between each vertebra.

Evolutionary Variation

Extant African apes have three and four lumbar vertebrae (Bonobos have different spines with an additional vertebra) and modern humans normally five. This difference, and because the lumbar spines of *Nacholapithecus* (a Miocene hominoid with six lumbar vertebrae and no tail) are similar to those of early *Australopithecus* and early *Homo*, it can be assumed that the Chimpanzee-human last common ancestor (PHLCA) also had a long axial column with a long lumbar region, and that the reduction in the number of lumbar vertebrae occurred independently in each ape clade. The limited number of lumbar vertebrae in chimpanzees and gorillas result in an inability to lordose their lumbar spines, in contrast to the spines of Old World monkeys and *Nacholapithecus* and *Proconsul*, which suggests that the PHLCA was not "short-backed" as previously believed.

Sacrum

In humans, the sacrum (plural: *sacrums* or *sacra*) is a large, triangular bone at the base of the spine and at the upper and back part of the pelvic cavity, where it is inserted like a wedge between the two hip bones. Its upper part connects with the last lumbar vertebra, and bottom part with the coccyx (tailbone). It consists of usually five initially unfused vertebrae which begin to fuse between ages 16–18 and are usually completely fused into a single bone by age 34. It is curved upon itself and placed obliquely (that is, tilted forward). It is kyphotic

— that is, concave facing forwards. The base projects forward as the sacral promontory internally, and articulates with the last lumbar vertebra to form the prominent sacrovertebral angle. The central part is curved outward towards the posterior, allowing greater room for the pelvic cavity. The two lateral projections of the sacrum are called ala (wings), and articulate with the ilium at the L-shaped sacroiliac joints.

Etymology

The name is derived from the Latin *(os) sacrum*, (*sacer, sacra, sacrum*, "sacred"), a translation of the Greek *hieron (osteon)*, meaning sacred or strong bone. Since the sacrum is the seat of the organs of procreation, animal sacra were offered in sacrifices. In Slavic languages and in German this bone is called the 'cross bone' (Kreuzbein), in Dutch 'holy bone' (Heiligbeen).

Parts

- The pelvic surface of the sacrum is concave from above downward, and slightly so from side to side.
- The dorsal surface of the sacrum is convex and narrower than the pelvic.
- The lateral surface of the sacrum is broad above, but narrowed into a thin edge below.
- The base of the sacrum, which is broad and expanded, is directed upward and forward.
- The apex (*apex oss. sacri*) is directed downward, and presents an oval facet for articulation with the coccyx.
- The vertebral canal (*canalis sacralis*; sacral canal) runs throughout the greater part of the bone; above, it is triangular in form; below, its posterior wall is incomplete, from the non-development of the laminae and spinous processes. It lodges the sacral nerves, and its walls are perforated by the anterior and posterior sacral foramina through which these nerves pass out.

Articulations

The sacrum articulates with four bones:

- the last lumbar vertebra above
- the coccyx (tailbone)

Rotation of the sacrum forward a few degrees vis-à-vis the ilia is sometimes called "nutation" (from the Latin term nutatio which means "nodding"), and the reverse (posterior) motion "counter-nutation." In upright vertebrates, the sacrum is capable of slight independent movement along the sagittal plane. When you bend backward the top (base) of the sacrum moves forward relative to the ilium; when you bend forward the top moves back. The *sacrum* is called so when referred to all of the parts combined. Its parts are called *sacral vertebrae* when referred individually.

Sexual Dimorphism

The sacrum is noticeably sexually dimorphic (differently-shaped in males and females). In the female the sacrum is shorter and wider than in the male; the lower half forms a greater angle with the upper; the upper half is nearly straight, the lower half presenting the greatest amount of curvature. The bone is also directed more obliquely backward; this increases the size of the pelvic cavity and renders the sacrovertebral angle more prominent. In the male the curvature is more evenly distributed over the whole length of the bone, and is altogether larger than in the female.

Variations

In some cases the sacrum will consist of six pieces [1] or be reduced in number to four [2]. The bodies of the first and second vertebrae may fail to unite. Sometimes the uppermost transverse tubercles are not joined to the rest of the ala on one or both sides, or the sacral canal may be open throughout a considerable part of its length, in consequence of the imperfect development of the laminae and spinous processes. The sacrum also varies considerably with respect to its degree of curvature.

Coccyx

The coccyx, commonly referred to as the tailbone, is the final segment of the vertebral column in tailless primates. Comprising three to five separate or fused vertebrae (the coccygeal vertebrae) below the sacrum, it is attached to the sacrum by a fibrocartilaginous joint, the sacrococcygeal symphysis, which permits limited movement between the sacrum and the coccyx. The term *coccyx* comes originally from the Greek "cuckoo", referring to the curved shape of a cuckoo's beak when viewed from the side.

Function

In humans and other tailless primates (e.g., great apes) since *Nacholapithecus* (a Miocene hominoid), the coccyx is the remnant of a vestigial tail, but still not entirely useless; it is an important attachment for various muscles, tendons and ligaments—which makes it necessary for physicians and patients to pay special attention to these attachments when considering surgical removal of the coccyx.

Additionally, it is also a part of the weight-bearing tripod structure which acts as a support for a sitting person. When a person sits leaning forward, the ischial tuberosities and inferior rami of the ischium take most of the weight, but as the sitting person leans backward, more weight is transferred to the coccyx.

The anterior side of the coccyx serves for the attachment of a group of muscles important for many functions of the pelvic floor (i.e., defecation, continence, etc.): The levator ani muscle, which include coccygeus, iliococcygeus, and pubococcygeus. Through the anococcygeal raphé, the coccyx supports the position of the anus. Attached to the posterior side is gluteus maximus which extend the thigh during ambulation.

Many important ligaments attach to the coccyx: The anterior and posterior sacrococcygeal ligaments are the continuations of the anterior and posterior longitudinal ligaments that stretches along the entire spine. Additionally, the lateral sacrococcygeal ligaments complete the foramina for the last sacral nerve. And, lastly, some fibres of the sacrospinous and sacrotuberous ligaments (arising from the spine of the ischium and the ischial tuberosity respectively) also attach to the coccyx. An extension of the pia mater, the filum terminale, extends from the apex of the conus, and inserts on the coccyx.

Structure

The coccyx is usually formed of four rudimentary vertebrae (sometimes five or three). It articulates superiorly with the sacrum. In each of the first three segments may be traced a rudimentary body and articular and transverse processes; the last piece (sometimes the third) is a mere nodule of bone. The transverse processes are most prominent and noticeable on the first coccygeal segment. All the segments are destitute of pedicles, laminae and spinous processes. The first is the largest; it resembles the lowest sacral vertebra, and often exists as a separate piece; the last three diminish in size from above downward. Most anatomy books wrongly state that the coccyx is normally fused in adults. In fact it has been shown that the coccyx may consist of up to five separate bony segments, the most common configuration being two or three segments.

Surfaces

The anterior surface is slightly concave and marked with three transverse grooves that indicate the junctions of the different segments. It gives attachment to the anterior sacrococcygeal ligament and the Levatores ani and supports part of the rectum.

The posterior surface is convex marked by transverse grooves similar to those on the anterior surface, and presents on either side a linear row of tubercles, the rudimentary articular processes of the coccygeal vertebrae.

Of these, the superior pair are large, and are called the coccygeal cornua; they project upward, and articulate with the cornua of the sacrum, and on either side complete the foramen for the transmission of the posterior division of the fifth sacral nerve.

Borders

The lateral borders are thin and exhibit a series of small eminences, which represent the transverse processes of the coccygeal vertebrae. Of these, the first is the largest; it is flattened from before backward, and often ascends to join the lower part of the thin lateral edge of the sacrum, thus completing the foramen for the transmission of the anterior division of the fifth sacral nerve; the others diminish in size from above downward, and are often wanting. The borders of the coccyx are narrow, and give attachment on either side to the sacrotuberous and sacrospinous ligaments, to the coccygeus in front of the ligaments, and to the gluteus maximus behind them.

Apex: The apex is rounded, and has attached to it the tendon of the Sphincter ani externus. It may be bifid.

Sacrococcygeal and Intercoccygeal Joints: The joints are variable and may be: (1) synovial joints; (2) thin discs of fibrocartilage; (3) intermediate between these two; (4) ossified.

Pathology

Injuring the coccyx can give rise to a painful condition called coccydynia and one or more of the bones or the connections thereof may be broken, fractured tailbone. A number of tumors are known to involve the coccyx; of these, the most common is sacrococcygeal teratoma.

Both coccydynia and coccygeal tumors may require surgical removal of the coccyx (coccygectomy). One complication of cocygectomy is a coccygeal hernia. Fortunately, most cases of coccyx pain respond well to nonsurgical treatment, such as medications given by local injection (often done under fluoroscopic guidance).

Development

The striking segmented pattern of the human spine is established during embryogenesis when the precursor of the vertebrae, the somites, are rhythmically added to the forming posterior part of the embryo.

In humans, somite formation begins around the third week post-fertilization and continues until a total of around 52 somites are formed. The somites are epithelial spheres that contain the precursors of the vertebrae, the ribs, the skeletal muscles of the body wall and limbs, and the dermis of the back.

The periodicity of somite distribution and production is thought to be imposed by a molecular oscillator or clock acting in cells of the presomitic mesoderm (PSM). Somites form soon after the beginning of gastrulation, on both sides of the neural tube from a tissue called the presomitic mesoderm (PSM). The PSM is part of the paraxial mesoderm and is generated caudally by gastrulation when cells ingress through the primitive streak, and later, through the tail bud.

Soon after their formation, somites become subdivided into the dermomyotome dorsally, which gives rise to the muscles and dermis, and the sclerotome ventrally, which will form the spine components. Sclerotomes become subdivided into an anterior and a posterior compartment.

This subdivision plays a key role in the definitive patterning of vertebrae that form when the posterior part of one somite fuses to the anterior part of the consecutive somite during a process termed resegmentation. Disruption of the somitogenesis process in humans results in diseases such as congenital scoliosis. So far, the human homologues of three genes associated to the mouse segmentation clock (MESP2, DLL3 and LFNG) have been shown to be mutated in human patients with human congenital scoliosis suggesting that the mechanisms involved in vertebral segmentation are conserved across vertebrates.

In humans the first four somites are incorporated in the basi-occipital bone of the skull and the next 33 somites will form the vertebrae. The remaining posterior somites degenerate. During the fourth week of embryonic development, the sclerotomes shift their position to surround the spinal cord and the notochord. The sclerotome is made of mesoderm and originates from the ventromedial part of the somites. This column of tissue has a segmented appearance, with alternating areas of dense and less dense areas.

As the sclerotome develops, it condenses further eventually developing into the vertebral body. Development of the appropriate shapes of the vertebral bodies is regulated by *HOX genes*. The less dense tissue that separates the sclerotome segments develop into the intervertebral discs. The notochord disappears in the sclerotome (vertebral body) segments, but persists in the region of the intervertebral discs as the nucleus pulposus. The nucleus pulposus and the fibres of the annulus fibrosus make up the intervertebral disc.

There are various defects associated with vertebral development. Scoliosis will result in improper fusion of the vertebrae. In Klippel-Feil anomaly patients have two or more cervical vertebrae that are fused together, along with other associated birth defects. One of the most serious defects is failure of the vertebral arches to fuse. This results in a condition called spina bifida. There are several variations of spina bifida that reflect the severity of the defect. The primary curves (thoracic and sacral curvatures) form during fetal development. The secondary curves develop after birth. The cervical curvature forms as a result of lifting the head and the lumbar curvature forms as a result of walking.

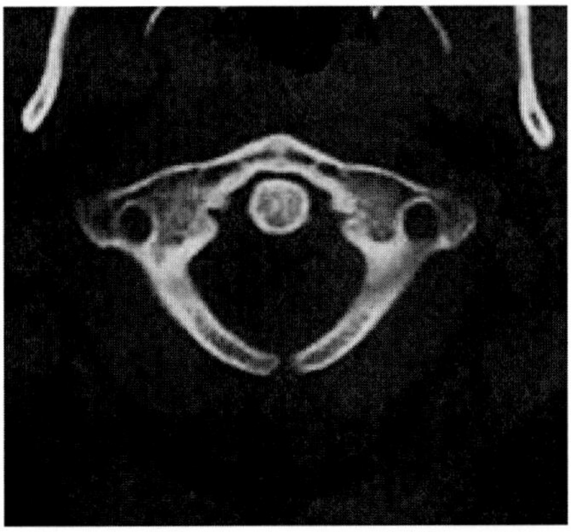

Figure: *Unfused arch of C1 at CT.*

Surfaces

Anterior Surface: When viewed from in front, the width of the bodies of the vertebrae is seen to increase from the second cervical to the first thoracic; there is then a slight diminution in the next three vertebrae; below this there is again a gradual and progressive increase in width as low as the sacrovertebral angle. From this point there is a rapid diminution, to the apex of the coccyx.

Posterior Surface

The posterior surface of the vertebral column presents in the median line the spinous processes. In the cervical region (with the exception of the second and seventh vertebrae) these are short and horizontal, with bifid extremities. In the upper part of the thoracic region they are directed obliquely downward; in the middle they are almost vertical, and in the lower part they are nearly horizontal. In the lumbar region they are nearly horizontal. The spinous processes are separated by considerable intervals in the lumbar region, by narrower intervals in the neck, and are closely approximated in the middle of the thoracic region. Occasionally one of these processes deviates a little from the median line — a fact to be remembered in practice, as irregularities of this sort are attendant also on fractures or displacements of the vertebral column.

On either side of the spinous processes is the vertebral groove formed by the laminae in the cervical and lumbar regions, where it is shallow, and by the laminae and transverse processes in the thoracic region, where it is deep and broad; these grooves lodge the deep muscles of the back. Lateral to the vertebral grooves are the articular processes, and still more laterally the transverse processes.

In the thoracic region, the transverse processes stand backward, on a plane considerably behind that of the same processes in the cervical and lumbar regions. In the cervical region, the transverse processes are placed in front of the articular processes, lateral to the pedicles and between the intervertebral foramina. In the thoracic region they are posterior to the pedicles, intervertebral foramina, and articular processes. In the lumbar region they are in front of the articular processes, but behind the intervertebral foramina.

Lateral Surfaces

The lateral surfaces are separated from the posterior surface by the articular processes in the cervical and lumbar regions, and by the transverse processes in the thoracic region. They present, in back, the sides of the bodies of the vertebrae, marked in the thoracic region by the facets for articulation with the heads of the ribs. More posteriorly are the intervertebral foramina, formed by the juxtaposition of the vertebral notches, oval in shape, smallest in the cervical and upper part of the thoracic regions, and gradually increasing in size to the last lumbar. They transmit the special spinal nerves and are situated between the transverse processes in the cervical region, and in front of them in the thoracic and lumbar regions.

Vertebral Canal

The vertebral canal follows the different curves of the column; it is large and triangular in those parts of the column which enjoy the greatest freedom of movement, such as the cervical and lumbar regions; and is small and rounded in the thoracic region, where motion is more limited.

Abnormalities

Occasionally the coalescence of the laminae is not completed, and consequently a cleft is left in the arches of the vertebrae, through which a protrusion of the spinal membranes (*dura mater* and arachnoid), and generally of the spinal cord (*medulla spinalis*) itself, takes place, constituting the malformation known as *spina bifida*. This condition is most common in the lumbosacral region, but it may occur in the thoracic or cervical region, or the arches throughout the whole length of the canal may remain incomplete.

The Following Abnormal Curvatures may Occur in Some People:

- Kyphosis is an exaggerated kyphotic (posterior) curvature in the thoracic region. This produces the so-called "humpback" or "dowager's hump", a condition commonly observed in osteoporosis.
- Lordosis is an exaggerated lordotic (anterior) curvature of the lumbar region, "swayback". Temporary lordosis is common among pregnant women.
- Retrolisthesis is a posterior displacement of one vertebral body with respect to the adjacent vertebral segment to a degree less than a luxation (dislocation).
- Scoliosis, lateral curvature, is the most common abnormal curvature, occurring in 0.5% of the population. It is more common among females and may result from unequal growth of the two sides of one or more vertebrae. It can also be caused by pulmonary atelectasis (partial or complete deflation of one or more lobes of the lungs) as observed in asthma or pneumothorax.

In Other Animals

In animals, vertebrae are defined by the regions of the vertebral column they occur in. Cervical vertebrae are those in the neck area. With exception of two sloth genera (*Choleopus* and *Bradypus*) and the manatee (*Trichechus*), all mammals have seven cervical vertebrate. In other vertebrates it can range from a single vertebra in amphibians, to as many as 25 in swans or 76 in the extinct plesiosaur *Elasmosaurus*. The dorsal vertebrae range from the bottom of the neck to the top of the pelvis. Dorsal vertebrae attached to ribs are called thoracic vertebrae, while those without ribs are called lumbar vertebrae. The sacral vertebrae are those in the pelvic region, and range from one in amphibians, to two in most birds and modern reptiles, or up to 3 to 5 in mammals. When multiple sacral vertebrae are fused into a single structure, it is called the sacrum. The synsacrum is a similar fused structure found in birds that is composed of the sacral, lumbar, and some of the thoracic and caudal vertebra, as well as the pelvic girdle. Caudal vertebrae compose the tail, and the final few can be fused into the pygostyle in birds, or into the coccygeal or tail bone in chimpanzees (and humans).

Structure of Individual Vertebrae

Individual vertebrae are composed of a centrum (body), arches protruding from the top and bottom of the centrum, and various processes projecting from the centrum and/or arches. An arch extending from the top of the centrum is called a neural arch, while the hemal arch or chevron is found underneath the centrum in the caudal (tail) vertebrae of fish, most reptiles, some birds, and some mammals with long tails. The vertebral processes can either give the structure rigidity, help them articulate with ribs, or serve as muscle attachment points. Common types are transverse process, diapophyses, parapophyses, and zygapophyses (both the cranial zygapophyses and the caudal zygapophyses).

Classification

The centra of the vertebra can be classified based upon the fusion of its elements. In aspidospondyly, bones such as the neural spine, the pleurocentrum and the intercentrum are separate ossifications. Fused elements, however, classify a vertebra as having holospondyly. A vertebra can also be described in terms of the shape of the ends of the centra. Centra with flat ends are *acoelous*, like those in mammals. These flat ends of the centra are especially good at supporting and distributing compressive forces. *Amphicoelous* vertebra have centra with both ends concave. This shape is common in fish, where most motion is limited. Amphicoelous centra often are integrated with a full notochord. *Procoelous* vertebrae are anteriorly concave and posteriorly convex. They are found in frogs and modern reptiles. *Opisthocoelous* vertebrae are the opposite, possessing anterior convexity and posterior concavity. They are found in salamanders. *Heterocoelous* vertebrae have saddle-shaped articular surfaces. This type of configuration is seen in turtles that retract their necks, and birds, because it permits extensive lateral and vertical flexion motion without stretching the nerve cord too extensively or wringing it about its long axis.

Fish and Amphibians

The vertebrae of lobe-finned fishes consist of three discrete bony elements. The vertebral arch surrounds the spinal cord, and is of broadly similar form to that found in most other vertebrates. Just beneath the arch lies a small plate-like pleurocentrum, which protects the upper surface of the notochord, and below that, a larger arch-shaped intercentrum to protect the lower border.

Both of these structures are embedded within a single cylindrical mass of cartilage. A similar arrangement was found in the primitive Labyrinthodonts, but in the evolutionary line that led to reptiles (and hence, also to mammals and birds), the intercentrum became partially or wholly replaced by an enlarged pleurocentrum, which in turn became the bony vertebral body.

In most ray-finned fishes, including all teleosts, these two structures are fused with, and embedded within, a solid piece of bone superficially resembling the vertebral body of mammals. In living amphibians, there is simply a cylindrical piece of bone below the vertebral arch, with no trace of the separate elements present in the early tetrapods.

In cartilagenous fish, such as sharks, the vertebrae consist of two cartilagenous tubes. The upper tube is formed from the vertebral arches, but also includes additional cartilagenous structures filling in the gaps between the vertebrae, and so enclosing the spinal cord in an essentially continuous sheath. The lower tube surrounds the notochord, and has a complex structure, often including multiple layers of calcification.

Lampreys have vertebral arches, but nothing resembling the vertebral bodies found in all higher vertebrates. Even the arches are discontinuous, consisting of separate pieces of arch-shaped cartilage around the spinal cord in most parts of the body, changing to long strips of cartilage above and below in the tail region. Hagfishes lack a true vertebral column, and are therefore not properly considered vertebrates, but a few tiny neural arches are present in the tail.

Amniotes

The general structure of human vertebrae is fairly typical of that found in mammals, reptiles, and birds. The shape of the vertebral body does, however, vary somewhat between different groups. In mammals, such as humans, it typically has flat upper and lower surfaces, while in reptiles the anterior surface commonly has a concave socket into which the expanded convex face of the next vertebral body fits.

Even these patterns are only generalisations, however, and there may be variation in form of the vertebrae along the length of the spine even within a single species. Some unusual variations include the saddle-shaped sockets between the cervical vertebrae of birds and the presence of a narrow hollow canal running down the centre of the vertebral bodies of geckos and tuataras, containing a remnant of the notochord.

Reptiles often retain the primitive intercentra, which are present as small crescent-shaped bony elements lying between the bodies of adjacent vertebrae; similar structures are often found in the caudal vertebrae of mammals. In the tail, these are attached to chevron-shaped bones called haemal arches, which attach below the base of the spine, and help to support the musculature. These latter bones are probably homologous with the ventral ribs of fish. The number of vertebrae in the spines of reptiles is highly variable, and may be several hundred in some species of snake.

In birds, there is a variable number of cervical vertebrae, which often form the only truly flexible part of the spine. The thoracic vertebrae are partially fused, providing a solid brace for the wings during flight.

The sacral vertebrae are fused with the lumbar vertebrae, and some thoracic and caudal vertebrae, to form a single structure, the synsacrum, which is thus of greater relative length than the sacrum of mammals. In living birds, the remaining caudal vertebrae are fused into a further bone, the pygostyle, for attachment of the tail feathers.

Aside from the tail, the number of vertebrae in mammals is generally fairly constant. There are almost always seven cervical vertebrae (sloths and manatees are among the few exceptions), followed by around twenty or so further vertebrae, divided between the thoracic and lumbar forms, depending on the number of ribs. There are generally three to five vertebrae with the sacrum, and anything up to fifty caudal vertebrae.

Notochord

The notochord is a flexible rod-shaped body found in embryos of all chordates. It is composed of cells derived from the mesoderm and defines the primitive axis of the embryo. In some chordates, it persists throughout life as the main axial support of the body, while in most vertebrates it becomes the nucleus pulposus of the intervertebral disc. The notochord is found ventral to the neural tube. Notochords were the first "backbones" serving as support structures in chordates such as *Haikouichthys*. Notochords were advantageous to primitive fish-ancestors because they were a rigid structure for muscle attachment, yet flexible enough to allow more movement than, for example, the exoskeleton of the dominant animals of that time. Embryos of vertebrates have notochords today, as it retained a key role in signalling and coordinating development even as it was lost in most adults. In most tetrapods, they eventually develop into the nucleus pulposus of the intervertebral discs.

Development of the Notochord

Notogenesis is the development of the notochord by the epiblasts that make up the floor of the amnion cavity (Human Embryology). The notochord arises from the bilaminar embryonic disk. The notochord forms during gastrulation and soon after induces the formation of the neural plate (neurulation), synchronizing the development of the neural tube.

On the ventral aspect of the neural groove an axial thickening of the endoderm takes place. (In bi-pedal chordates, e.g. humans, this surface is properly referred to as the anterior surface).

This thickening appears as a furrow (the chordal furrow) the margins of which anastomose (come into contact), and so convert it into a solid rod of polygonal-shaped cells (the notochord) which is then separated from the endoderm.

It extends throughout the entire length of the future vertebral column, and reaches as far as the anterior end of the midbrain, where it ends in a hook-like extremity in the region of the future dorsum sellæ of the sphenoid bone. Initially it exists between the neural tube and the endoderm of the yolk-sac, but soon becomes separated from them by the mesoderm, which grows medially and surrounds it. From the mesoderm surrounding the neural tube and notochord, the skull, vertebral column, and the membranes of the brain and medulla spinalis are developed.

Postembryonic vestige of the notochord is found in the nucleus pulposus of the intervertebral disks, but not in the vertebral bodies, from which notochordal cells usually regress entirely. In humans, by the age of 4, all notochord residue is replaced by a population of chondrocyte-like cells of unclear origin. Persistence of notochordal cells within the vertebra may cause a pathologic condition- persistent notochordal canal. They are also found to persist in the nasopharyngeal space and, in such an unusual instance, may give rise to Tornwaldt's cyst.

The Notochord in Neural Development

Research into the notochord has played a key role in understanding the development of the central nervous system. By transplanting and expressing a second notochord near the dorsal neural tube, 180 degrees opposite of the normal notochord location, one can induce the formation of motoneurons in the dorsal tube. Motoneuron formation generally occurs in the ventral neural tube, while the dorsal tube generally forms sensory cells. The notochord secretes a protein called sonic hedgehog homolog (SHH), a key morphogen regulating organogenesis and having a critical role in signaling the development of motoneurons. The secretion of SHH by the notochord establishes the ventral pole of the dorsal-ventral axis in the developing embryo.

Evolution of the Notochord

The notochord is the defining feature of Chordates, and was present throughout life in many of the earliest chordates. Although the stomochord of hemichordates was once thought to be homologous, it is now viewed as a convergence. Pikaia appears to have a proto-notochord, and notochords are present in several basal chordates such as Haikouella, Haikouichthys, and Myllokunmingia, all from the Cambrian.

The Ordovician oceans included many diverse species of agnathan fish which possessed notochords, either with attached bony elements or without, most notably the conodonts, placoderms and ostracoderms. Even after the evolution of the vertebral column in chondrichthyes and osteichthyes, these taxa remained common and are well represented in the fossils record. Several species have reverted to the primitive state, retaining the notochord into adulthood, though the reasons for this are not well-understood.

The Structure of the Notochord

The notochord is composed primarily of a core of glycoproteins, encased in a sheath of collagen fibres wound into two opposing helices. The angle between these fibres determines whether increased pressure in the core will result in shortening and thickening versus lengthening and thinning.

Chapter 3

Comparative Vertebrates

Vertebrate

Vertebrates are animals that are members of the subphylum Vertebrata /-QĐ/ (chordates with backbones and spinal columns). Vertebrates include the overwhelming majority of the phylum Chordata, with currently about 64,000 species described. Vertebrates include the jawless fish, bony fish, sharks and rays, amphibians, reptiles, mammals, and birds. Extant vertebrates range in size from the frog species *Paedophryne amauensis*, at as little as 7.7 mm (0.3 inch), to the blue whale, at up to 33 m (110 ft). Vertebrates make up about 4% of all described animal species; the rest are invertebrates, which lack backbones. The vertebrates traditionally include the hagfishes, which do not have proper vertebrae, though their closest living relatives, the lampreys, do have vertebrate. Hagfishes do, however, possess a cranium. For this reason, the vertebrate subphylum is sometimes referred to as "Craniata" when discussing morphology. Molecular analysis since 1992 has suggested that the hagfishes are most closely related to lampreys, and so also are vertebrates in a monophyletic sense. Others consider them a sister group of vertebrates in the common taxon of Craniata.

Etymology

The word *vertebrate* derives from the Latin word *vertebratus* (Pliny), meaning *joint of the spine*. It is closely related to the word *vertebra*, which refers to any of the bones or segments of the spinal column.

Anatomy and Morphology

All vertebrates are built along the basic chordate body plan: a stiff rod running through the length of the animal (vertebral column or notochord), with a hollow tube of nervous tissue (the spinal cord) above it and the gastrointestinal tract below. In all vertebrates, the mouth is found at, or right below, the anterior end of the animal, while the anus opens to the exterior before the end of the body. The remaining part of the body continuing aft of the anus forms a tail with vertebrae and spinal cord, but no gut.

Vertebral Column

The defining characteristic of a vertebrate is the vertebral column, in which the notochord (a stiff rod of uniform composition) found in all chordates has been replaced by a segmented series of stiffer elements (vertebrae) separated by mobile joints (intervertebral discs, derived embryonically and evolutionarily from the notochord). However, a few vertebrates have secondarily lost this anatomy, retaining the notochord into adulthood, such as the sturgeon and the *Latimeria.* Jawed vertebrates are typified by paired appendages (fins or legs, which may be secondarily lost), but this is not part of the definition of vertebrates as a whole.

Gills

All basal vertebrates breathe with gills. The gills are carried right behind the head, bordering the posterior margins of a series of openings from the esophagus to the exterior. Each gill is supported by a cartilagenous or bony gill arch. The bony fish have three pairs of arches, cartilaginous fish have five to seven pairs, while the primitive jawless fish have seven. The vertebrate ancestor no doubt had more arches, as some of their chordate relatives have more than 50 pairs of gills.

In amphibians and some primitive bony fishes, the larvae bear external gills, branching off from the gill arches. These are reduced in adulthood, their function taken over by the gills proper in fishes and by lungs in most amphibians. Some amphibans retain the external larval gills in adulthood, the complex internal gill system as seen in fish apparently being irrevocably lost very early in the evolution of tetrapods.

While the higher vertebrates do not have gills, the gill arches form during fetal development, and lay the basis of essential structures such as jaws, the thyroid gland, the larynx, the *columella* (corresponding to the stapes in mammals) and in mammals the malleus and incus.

Central Nervous System

The vertebrates are the only chordate group to exhibit a proper brain. A slight swelling of the anterior end of the nerve cord is found in the lancelet, though it lacks the eyes and other complex sense organs comparable to those of vertebrates. Other chordates do not show any trends towards cephalisation.

The central nervous system is based on a hollow nerve tube running along the length of the animal, from which the peripheral nervous system branches out to enervate the various systems. The front end of the nerve tube is expanded by a thickening of the walls and expansion of the central canal of spinal cord into three primary brain vesicles: The prosencephalon (forebrain), mesencephalon (midbrain) and rhombencephalon (hindbrain), further differentiated in the various vertebrate groups. Two laterally placed eyes form around outgrows from the midbrain, except in hagfish, though this may be a secondary loss. The forebrain is well developed and subdivided in most tetrapods, while the midbrain dominate in many fish and some salamanders. Vesicles of the forebrain are usually paired, giving rise to hemispheres like the cerebral hemispheres in mammals. The resulting anatomy of the central nervous system, with a single, hollow nerve cord topped by a series of (often paired) vesicles is unique to vertebrates. All invertebrates with well developed brains, like insects, spiders and squids have a ventral rather than dorsal system of ganglions, with a split brain stem running on each side of the mouth/gut.

Evolutionary History

First Vertebrates

Vertebrates originated about 525 million years ago during the Cambrian explosion, which saw the rise in organism diversity. The earliest known vertebrate is believed to be the *Myllokunmingia*. Another early vertebrate is *Haikouichthys ercaicunensis*. Unlike the other fauna that dominated the

Cambrian, these groups had the basic vertebrate body plan: a notochord, rudimentary vertebrae, and a well-defined head and tail. All of these early vertebrates lacked jaws in the common sense and relied on filter feeding close to the seabed.

From Fish to Amphibians

The first jawed vertebrates appeared in the latest Ordovician and became common in the Devonian, often known as the "Age of Fishes". The two groups of bony fishes, the actinopterygii and sarcopterygii, evolved and became common. The Devonian also saw the demise of virtually all jawless fishes, save for lampreys and hagfish, as well as the Placodermi, a group of armoured fish that dominated much of the late Silurian. The Devonian also saw the rise of the first labyrinthodonts, which was a transitional between fishes and amphibians.

Mesozoic Vertebrates

The reptiles appeared from labyrinthodonts in the subsequent Carboniferous period. The anapsid and synapsid reptiles were common during the late Paleozoic, while the diapsids became dominant during the Mesozoic. In the sea, the bony fishes became dominant. The dinosaurs gave rise to the birds in the Jurassic. The demise of the dinosaurs at the end of the Cretaceous promoted expansion of the mammals, which had evolved from the therapsids, a group of synapsid reptiles, during the late Triassic Period.

After the Mesozoic

The Cenozoic world has seen great diversification of bony fishes, frogs, birds and mammals. Over half of all living vertebrate species (about 32,000 species) are fishes (non-tetrapod craniates), a diverse set of lineages that inhabit all the world's aquatic ecosystems, from snow minnows (Cypriniformes) in Himalayan lakes at elevations over 4,600 metres (15,000 feet) to flatfishes (order Pleuronectiformes) in the Challenger Deep, the deepest ocean trench at about 11,000 metres (36,000 feet). Fishes of myriad varieties are the main predators in most of the world's water bodies, both freshwater and marine. The rest of the vertebrate species are tetrapods, a single lineage that includes amphibians (frogs, with more than 5,800 species; salamanders, with about 580 species; and caecilians, with about

175 species); mammals (with over 5,400 species); and reptiles and birds (with more than 18,000 species).

Tetrapods dominate the megafauna of most terrestrial environments (including fossorial and arboreal realms) and also include many partially or fully aquatic groups (e.g., sea snakes, penguins, cetaceans).

Classification

There are several ways of classifying animals. Evolutionary systematics relies on anatomy, physiology and evolutionary history, which is determined through similarities in anatomy and, if possible, the genetics of organisms. Phylogenetic classification is based solely on phylogeny. Evolutionary systematics gives an overview; phylogenetic systematics gives detail. The two systems are thus complementary rather than opposed. Conventional classification has living vertebrates grouped into seven classes based on traditional interpretations of gross anatomical and physiological traits. This classification is the one most commonly encountered in school textbooks, overviews, non-specialist, and popular works. The extant vertebrates are:

- Subphylum Vertebrata
  - Class Agnatha (jawless fishes)
  - Class Chondrichthyes (cartilaginous fishes)
  - Class Osteichthyes (bony fishes)
  - Class Amphibia (amphibians)
  - Class Reptilia (reptiles)
  - Class Aves (birds)
  - Class Mammalia (mammals).

In addition to these comes two classes of extinct armoured fishes, the Placodermi and the Acanthodii. Other ways of classifying the vertebrates have been devised, particularly with emphasis on the phylogeny on early amphibians and reptiles. An example based on Janvier (1981, 1997), Shu *et al.* (2003), and Benton (2004) is given here:

- Subphylum Vertebrata
  - Superclass Agnatha or Cephalaspidomorphi (lampreys and other jawless fishes)

- Infraphylum Gnathostomata (vertebrates with jaws)
  - Class †Placodermi (extinct armoured fishes)
  - Class Chondrichthyes (cartilaginous fishes)
  - Class †Acanthodii (extinct spiny "sharks")
  - Superclass Osteichthyes (bony fishes)
  - Class Actinopterygii (ray-finned bony fishes)
  - Class Sarcopterygii (lobe-finned fishes, some ancestral to tetrapods)
  - Superclass Tetrapoda (four-limbed vertebrates)
  - Class Amphibia (amphibians, some ancestral to the amniotes)
  - Class †Synapsida (extinct mammal-like "reptiles", some ancestral to mammals, sometimes classed with Reptilia)
  - Class Reptilia (reptiles, some ancestral to birds)
  - Class Aves (birds)
  - Class Mammalia (mammals).

While this traditional classification is orderly, most of the groups are paraphyletic, i.e. do not contain all descendants of the class's common ancestor.

For instance, descendants of the first reptiles include modern reptiles as well as birds. Most of the classes listed are not "complete" taxa, meaning that they do not include all the descendants of the first representative of the group.

For example, the agnathans have given rise to the jawed vertebrates; the bony fishes have given rise to the land vertebrates; the traditional "amphibians" have given rise to the reptiles (traditionally including the synapsids, or "mammal-like "reptiles"), which in turn have given rise to the mammals and birds.

Most scientists working with vertebrates use a classification based purely on phylogeny, organised by their known evolutionary history and sometimes disregarding the conventional interpretations of their anatomy and physiology.

Phylogenetic Relationships

In phylogenetic taxonomy, the relationships between animals are not typically divided into ranks, but illustrated as a nested "family tree" known as a cladogram. Phylogenetic groups are given definitions based on their relationship to one another, rather than purely on physical traits such as the presence of a backbone. This nesting pattern is often combined with traditional taxonomy (as above), in a practice known as evolutionary taxonomy.

Chordate

Chordates, members of the phylum Chordata, are deuterostome animals possessing a notochord, a hollow dorsal nerve cord, pharyngeal slits, an endostyle, and a post-anal tail for at least some period of their life cycles. Taxonomically, the phylum includes the subphyla Vertebrata, including mammals (and thus humans), fish, amphibians, reptiles, birds; Tunicata, including salps and sea squirts; and Cephalochordata, comprising the lancelets.

The phylum Hemichordata including the acorn worms has been presented as a fourth chordate subphylum, but it now is usually treated as a separate phylum. It, along with the echinoderm phylum, including starfish, sea urchins, and sea cucumbers and their kin, are the chordates' closest relatives. Primitive chordates are known from at least as early as the Cambrian explosion. There are more than 60,000 living species of chordates, about half of which are bony fish of the class osteichthyes. The world's largest animal, the blue whale, and fastest animal, the peregrine falcon, are chordates.

Overview of Affinities

Tunicate larvae have both a notochord and a nerve cord which are lost in adulthood. Cephalochordates have a notochord and a nerve cord (but no brain or specialist sensory organs) and a very simple circulatory system. Craniates are the only subphylum whose members have skulls. In all craniates except for hagfish, the dorsal hollow nerve cord is surrounded with cartilaginous or bony vertebrae and the notochord is generally reduced; hence, hagfish are not universally regarded as vertebrates, though recent DNA comparisons suggest that they are in fact vertebrates. The chordates and three sister phyla, the Hemichordata, the Echinodermata and the Xenoturbellida, make up the deuterostomes, one of the two superphyla that encompass all fairly complex animals. Attempts to work out the evolutionary relationships of the chordates have produced several hypotheses. The current consensus is that chordates are monophyletic, meaning that the Chordata include all and only the descendants of a single common ancestor *which is itself a chordate*, and that craniates' nearest relatives are cephalochordates. All of the earliest chordate fossils have been found in the Early Cambrian Chengjiang fauna, and include two species that are regarded as fish, which implies they are vertebrates. Because the fossil record of chordates is poor, only molecular phylogenetics offers a reasonable prospect of dating their emergence. However, the use of molecular phylogenetics for dating evolutionary transitions is controversial.

It has also proved difficult to produce a detailed classification within the living chordates. Attempts to produce evolutionary "family trees" give results that differ from traditional classes because several of those classes are not monophyletic. As a result, vertebrate classification is in a state of flux.

Origin of Name

Although the name Chordata is often attributed to William Bateson (1885), it was already in prevalent use in by 1880. Ernst Haeckel described a taxon comprising tunicates, cephalochordates, and vertebrates in 1866. Though he used the German vernacular form, it is allowed under the ICZN code because of its subsequent latinization.

Definition

Chordates form a phylum of creatures that are based on a bilateral body plan, and is defined by having at some stage in their lives all of the following:

- A notochord, in other words a fairly stiff rod of cartilage that extends along the inside of the body. Among the vertebrate sub-group of chordates the notochord develops into the spine, and in wholly aquatic species this helps the animal to swim by flexing its tail.

- A dorsal neural tube. In fish and other vertebrates this develops into the spinal cord, the main communications trunk of the nervous system.
- Pharyngeal slits. The pharynx is the part of the throat immediately behind the mouth. In fish the slits are modified to form gills, but in some other chordates they are part of a filter-feeding system that extracts particles of food from the water in which the animals live.
- Post-anal tail. A muscular tail that extends backwards behind the anus.
- An endostyle. This is a groove in the ventral wall of the pharynx. In filter-feeding species it produces mucus to gather food particles, which helps in transporting food to the esophagus. It also stores iodine, and may be a precursor of the vertebrate thyroid gland.

Craniata

Craniata (sometimes Craniota) is a proposed clade of chordate animals that contains the Myxini (hagfish), Petromyzontida (including lampreys), and Gnathostomata (jawed vertebrates) as living representatives. As the name suggests, Craniata are animals with a (hard bone or cartilage) skull in Chordata.

Characteristics

In the simplest sense craniates are chordates with heads, thus excluding members of chordate subphyla Urochordata (tunicates) and Cephalochordata (lancelets), but including Myxini, which have cartilaginous skulls and tooth-like structures composed of keratin.

Craniata also includes all lampreys and armored jawless fishes, armoured fish, sharks, skates, and rays, and Teleostomians:spiny sharks, bony fish, lissamphibians, temnospondyls and protoreptiles, reptiles, birds and mammals. The craniate head consists of a brain, sense organs including eyes, and a skull.

In addition to distinct crania (sing. *cranium*), craniates possess many derived characteristics which have allowed for more complexity to follow. Molecular-genetic analysis of craniates reveals that, compared to less complex animals, they developed duplicate sets of many gene families that are involved in cell signaling, transcription, and morphogenesis.

In general, craniates are much more active than tunicates and lancelets and as a result have greater metabolic demands, as well as several anatomical adaptations. Aquatic craniates have gill slits which are connected to muscles and nerves which pump water through the slits (as opposed to lancelets, whose pharyngeal slits are used only for suspension feeding), engaging in both feeding and gas exchange.

Muscles line the alimentary canal, moving food through the canal, allowing higher craniates like mammals to develop more complex digestive systems for optimal food processing. Craniates have cardiovascular systems which include a heart with two or more chambers, red blood cells, and O_2 transporting hemoglobin, as well as kidneys.

Systematics and Taxonomy

Linnaeus (1758) used the terms 'Craniata' and 'Vertebrata' interchangeably to include lampreys, jawed fishes, and terrestrial vertebrates (tetrapods). Hagfishes were classified as Vermes, possibly representing a transitional form between 'worms' and fishes. Dumeril (1806) grouped hagfishes and lampreys in the taxon 'Cyclostomi', characterized by horny teeth borne on a tongue-like apparatus, a large notochord as adults, and pouch-shaped gills (Marspibranchii).

Cyclostomes were regarded as either degenerate cartilaginous fishes or primitive vertebrates. Cope (1889) coined the name 'Agnatha' (jawless) for a group that included the cyclostomes and a number of fossil groups in which jaws could not be observed. Vertebrates were subsequently divided into two major sister-groups; Agnatha and Gnathostomata (jawed vertebrates). Stensio (1927) suggested that the two groups of living agnathans (i.e., cyclostomes) arose independently from different groups of fossil agnathans. Løvtrup (1977) argued that lampreys are more closely related to gnathostomes based on a number of uniquely derived characters, including: arcualia (serially arranged paired cartilages above the notochord), extrinsic eyeball muscles, radial muscles in the fins, a closely set atrium and ventricle of the heart, nervous regulation of the heart (by the vagus nerve), a typhlosole (spirally coiled valve of the intestinal wall), true lymphocytes, a differentiated anterior lobe of the pituitary gland (adenohypophysis), three inner ear maculae (patches of acceleration sensitive 'hair cells' used in balance) organised into two or three vertical semicircular canals, neuromast organs (composed of vibration sensitive hair cells) in the laterosensory canals, an electroreceptive lateral line (with voltage sensitive hair cells) and electrosensory lateral line nerves, and a cerebellum (i.e., the multi-layered roof of the hindbrain with unique structure [characteristic neural architecture including direct inputs from the lateral line and large output Purkinje cells) and function [integrating sensory perception and coordinating motor control]).

In other words, the 'cyclostome' characteristics (e.g., horny teeth, "tongue", gill pouches) are either instances of convergent evolution for feeding and gill ventilation in animals with an eel-like body shape, or represent primitive craniate characteristics subsequently lost or modified in gnathostomes. Janvier (1978) proposed to use the names 'Vertebrata' and 'Craniata' as two distinct and nested taxa.

Validity

The validity of the taxon "Craniata" was recently examined by Delarbre et al. (2002) using mtDNA sequence data, concluding that Myxini is more closely related to Hyperoartia than to Gnathostomata - i.e., that modern jawless fishes form a clade called Cyclostomata. The argument is that if Craniata is indeed monophyletic, Vertebrata would return to its old content (Gnathostomata + Cyclostomata) and the name Craniata, being superfluous, would become a junior synonym.

The new evidence removes support for the hypothesis for the evolutionary sequence by which (from among tunicate-like chordates) first the hard cranium arose as it is exhibited by the hagfish, then the backbone as exhibited by the lampreys, and then finally the hinged jaw that is now ubiquitous. In 2010, Philippe Janvier stated: Although I was among the early supporters of vertebrate paraphyly, I am impressed by the evidence provided by Heimberg et al. and prepared to admit that cyclostomes are, in fact, monophyletic. The consequence is that they may tell us little, if anything, about the dawn of vertebrate evolution, except that the intuitions of 19th century zoologists were correct in assuming that these odd vertebrates (notably, hagûshes) are strongly degenerate and have lost many characters over time.

Tunicate

Tunicates, previously known as Urochordata or urochordates, are members of the Tunicata, a subphylum of the phylum Chordata. They are marine filter feeders with a saclike morphology. In their respiration and feeding they take in water through an incurrent (or inhalant) siphon and expel the filtered water through an excurrent (or exhalant) siphon.

Most adult tunicates are sessile and attached to rocks or similarly suitable surfaces on the ocean floor; others such as salps, doliolids and pyrosomes swim in the pelagic zone as adults. Various species are commonly known as sea squirts or sea pork. The Tunicata apparently evolved in the early Cambrian period. Despite their simple appearance, they are a sister subphylum to the Vertebrata.

General Physiology, Morphology, and Development

Like other chordates, tunicates have a notochord during their early development, but by the time they have completed their larval stages they have lost all myomeric segmentation throughout the body. As members of the Chordata they are true Coelomata with endoderm, ectoderm and mesoderm, but they do not develop very clear coelomic body-cavities if any at all. Whether they do or not, by the end of their larval development all that remain are the pericardial, renal, and gonadal cavities of the adults.

Except for the heart, gonads, and pharynx (or branchial sac), the organs are enclosed in a membrane called an epicardium, which is surrounded by the jelly-like mesenchyme. Tunicates begin life in a mobile larval stage that resembles a tadpole. A minority of species, those in the Larvacea, retain the general larval form throughout life, but most Tunicata very rapidly settle down and attach themselves to a suitable surface, later developing into a barrel-like and usually sedentary adult form. The Thaliacea however, are pelagic throughout their lives and their life cycles may be complex, as for example in the Salpida. Tunicates lack kidney-like metanephridial organs, but make do with a less elaborate nitrogenous excretory system. The typical renal organ is a mass of large clear-walled vesicles that occupy the rectal loop, and the structure has no duct. Each vesicle is a remnant of a part of the primitive coelom, and its cells extract nitrogenous waste matter from circulating blood. They accumulate the wastes inside the vesicles as urates and do not have any obvious means of disposing of the material during the life of the animal.

Tunicates are unusual among animals in that they produce a large fraction of their tunic and some other structures in the form of cellulose. Cellulose production in animals is so inconspicuous that some sources deny its presence outside plants, but for some time now it has been known to occur in the dermis of mammals. However, the Tunicata are unique in their scale of application and production of the material. When in 1845 Carl Schmidt first announced the presence in the test of some Ascidians of a substance very similar to cellulose, he called it "tunicine", but it now is recognised as cellulose rather than any alternative substance.

Feeding

Most tunicates are suspension feeders, capturing suspended particles and plankton by filtering sea water through their siphons via their pharyngeal slits, but some, such as the *Megalodicopia hians*, are marine sit-and-wait predators.

Tunicates have two openings in their body cavity: an incurrent and an excurrent siphon. The incurrent siphon takes in water plus any food it contains, and the excurrent siphon expels wastes plus sieved water. The primary food source for most tunicates is plankton that gets entangled in mucus secreted from the endostyle.

The tunicate's pharynx, or branchial sac, is lined with ciliated epithelium. The action of the cilia passes food particles and plankton down to the esophagus and also passes the stream of water from the inhalant to the exhalant siphon. The gut is U-shaped and also ciliated, and the anus opens into the dorsal or cloacal part of the peribranchial cavity near the atrial aperture, where the constant stream of water carries wastes to the exterior. Tunicate blood is particularly interesting. It contains high concentrations of the transition metal vanadium and vanadium-associated proteins as well as higher than usual levels of lithium. Some tunicates can concentrate vanadium up to a level one million times that of the surrounding seawater. Specialised cells can concentrate heavy metals, which are then deposited in the tunic.

Taxonomy

Urochordata is a junior synonym of Tunicata which was established by Lamarck in 1816. Balfour introduced the name Urochorda in 1881 in order to emphasize the affinity of the group to other chordates,. No doubt largely because of his influence, various authors supported the term, either as such, or as "Urochordata", but the usage is invalid because "Tunicata" has precedence and there never were grounds for superseding the name. Accordingly the current (formally correct) trend is to abandon the name Urochorda or Urochordata in favour of the original Tunicata, and the name Tunicata is almost invariably used in modern scientific works. It is accepted as valid by the World Register of Marine Species and by ITIS, the Integrated Taxonomic Information System.

The Tunicata Contains about 3,000 Species, Usually Divided into the Following Classes:

- Ascidiacea (Aplousobranchia, Phlebobranchia, and Stolidobranchia)
- Thaliacea (Pyrosomida, Doliolida, and Salpida)
- Appendicularia (Larvacea)
- Sorberacea.

Although the traditional classification is followed for now, newer evidence suggests that the Ascidiacea is an artificial group of paraphyletic status.

The new classification would be:

- Stolidobranchia
- Aplousobranchia, Phlebobranchia and Thaliacea
- Appendicularia
- Sorberacea would belong somewhere in Ascidiacea, or be in a taxon on its own.

The species *Ciona intestinalis* and *Ciona savignyi* have attracted interest in biology for developmental studies. Both species' mitochondrial and nuclear genomes have been sequenced. Moreover, the nuclear genome of the appendicularian *Oikopleura dioica* appears to be one of the smallest among metazoans. Sea squirts have become a testing ground in the controversy about the extent to which cross-species gene transfer and hybridization have influenced animal evolution.

In 1990, Donald I. Williamson of the University of Liverpool (U.K.) fertilised sea squirt (*Ascidia mentula*) eggs with sea urchin (*Echinus esculentus*) sperm resulting in fertile adults that resembled urchins, but Michael W. Hart of Simon Fraser University failed to find sea-squirt DNA in tissue samples from the supposed hybrids. Williamson claims to have repeated the experiment with sea urchin eggs and sea squirt sperm, producing sea urchin larvae which developed into squirt-like juveniles. On the other hand, Syvanen and Ducore of the University of California have suggested that sea squirts descended from a hybrid between a chordate and a likely extinct protostome ancestor at a time before the diversification of round worms and arthropods. This study also examined whether there was evidence of a sea urchin/tunicate hybridization event that could possibly explain the distribution of genes in modern sea squirts—none could be seen.

Life Cycle

Most tunicates are hermaphrodites. The eggs are kept inside their body until they hatch, while sperm is released into the water where it fertilizes other individuals when brought in with incoming water.

Some larval forms appear very much like primitive chordates with a notochord (stiffening rod). Superficially, the larva resemble small tadpoles. They swim with a tail, and may have a simple eye, or ocellus, and balancing organ, or statolith. Some forms have a calcareous spicule that may be preserved as a fossil. They have appeared from the Jurassic to the present, with one proposed Neoproterozoic form, *Yarnemia*.

The larval form ends when the tunicate finds a suitable rock to affix to and cements itself in place. The larval form is not capable of feeding, though it may have a digestive system, and is only a dispersal mechanism. Many physical changes occur to the tunicate's body, one of the most interesting being the digestion of the cerebral ganglion, which controls movement and is the equivalent of the human brain. From this comes the common saying that the sea squirt "eats its own brain". In some classes, the adults remain pelagic (swimming or drifting in the open sea), although their larvae undergo similar metamorphoses to a higher or lower degree.

In growing to adulthood, tunicates develop a thick protective covering, called a *tunic*, or *test*, around their barrel-shaped bodies. During embryonic development, tunicates exhibit "determinate cleavage", where the fate of the cells is set early on with reduced cell numbers and genomes that are rapidly evolving. In contrast, the amphioxus and vertebrates show cell determination relatively late in development and cell cleavage is indeterminate. The genome evolution of amphioxus and vertebrates is also relatively slow.

Fossil Record

Undisputed fossils of tunicates are rare. The best known (and earliest) is *Shankouclava shankouense* from the Lower Cambrian Maotianshan Shale at Shankou village, Anning, near Kunming (South China). There is also a common bioimmuration of a tunicate (*Catellocaula vallata*) found in Upper Ordovician bryozoan skeletons of the upper midwestern United States.

There are also two enigmatic species from the Ediacaran period - *Ausia fenestrata* from the Nama Group of Namibia and a second new *Ausia*-like genus from the Onega Peninsula, White Sea of northern Russia. Results of new study have shown possible affinity of these Ediacaran organisms to the ascidians. These two organisms lived in the shallow waters of a sea, slightly more than 555-548 million years ago and are likely the oldest evidence of the chordate lineage of metazoans. A Precambrian fossil known as *Yarnemia* has been referred to the Urochordata, however this assignment is doubtful. Complete body fossils of tunicates are rare, but in some tunicate families, microscopic spicules are generated which may be preserved as microfossils. Such spicules have occasionally been described from Jurassic and later rocks. Few paleontologists are familiar with them; tunicate spicules may be mistaken for sponge spicules.

Invasive Species

Over the past few years, urochordates (notably of the genera *Didemnum* and *Styela*) have been invading coastal waters in many countries, and are spreading quickly. The carpet tunicate (*Didemnum vexillum*) is a mat-like organism that can smother other sea life, has very few natural predators, and is causing much concern. *D. vexillum* colonies are yellowish cream in colour, and look like thick sponge-like masses and can overgrow objects on the sea floor such as gravel, mollusc shells, and possibly other encrusting species.

These colonies are flexible, irregular, long, flat, and often exist as branched outgrowths projected from the surface referred to as tendrils. Some of the tendrils result from the colony encrusting worm tubes or other cylindrical objects but many are solid with a firm gelatinous core. The individuals of the colony are called zooids and many zooids with individual siphonal openings cover the surface of the colony.

Introduction of invasive tunicates usually occurs by transport on the hulls of ships and possibly in ballast water. Current research indicates that many tunicates previously thought to be indigenous to Europe and the Americas are, in fact, invaders. Some of these invasions may have occurred centuries or even millennia ago. In some areas, tunicates are proving to be a major threat to aquaculture operations. The U.S. Geological Survey, NOAA Fisheries, and the University of Rhode Island are investigating this phenomenon as they have been spotted in 2004 in Georges Bank. They requested that any information or sightings of these invading colonies be reported to United States Geological Survey to aid in their investigation.

Medical Uses

Tunicates contain a host of potentially useful chemical compounds, including:

- Didemnins, effective against various types of cancer, as antivirals and immunosuppressants
- Aplidine, effective against various types of cancer
- Trabectedin, effective against various types of cancer.

In the May 2007 issue of The *FASEB* Journal, researchers from Stanford University showed that tunicates can correct abnormalities over a series of generations, and they suggest that a similar regenerative process may be possible for humans. The mechanisms underlying the phenomenon may lead to insights about the potential of cells and tissues to be reprogrammed and regenerate compromised human organs. Gerald Weissman, editor-in-chief of the journal, said "This study is a landmark in regenerative medicine; the Stanford group has accomplished the biological equivalent of turning a sow's ear into a silk purse and back again."

Lancelet

The lancelets (from "lancet"), also known as amphioxus, comprise some twenty-two species of fish-like marine chordates with a global distribution in shallow temperate (as far north as Scotland) and tropical seas, usually found half-buried in sand. They are the modern representatives of the subphylum Cephalochordata, formerly thought to be the sister group of the craniates. In Asia, they are harvested commercially as food for humans and domesticated animals.

They are an important object of study in zoology as they provide indications about the origins of the vertebrates. Lancelets serve as an intriguing comparison point for tracing how vertebrates have evolved and adapted.

Although lancelets split from vertebrates more than 520 million years ago, their genomes hold clues about evolution, particularly how vertebrates have employed old genes for new functions. They are regarded as similar to the archetypal vertebrate form. The genome of the Florida lancelet (*Branchiostoma floridae*) has been sequenced.

Physical Features

Lancelets grow up to about 5 centimetres (2.0 in) long, reaching 7 centimetres (2.8 in) at the longest. They have a translucent, somewhat fish-like body, but without any paired fins or other limbs. A relatively poorly developed tail fin is present, so they are not especially good swimmers. While they do possess some cartilage-like material stiffening the gill slits, mouth, and tail, they have no true skeleton.

In common with vertebrates, lancelets have a hollow nerve cord running along the back, pharyngeal slits and a tail that runs past the anus. Also like vertebrates, the muscles are arranged in blocks called myomeres.

Unlike vertebrates, the dorsal nerve cord is not protected by bone but by a simpler notochord made up of a cylinder of cells that are closely packed to form a toughened rod. The lancelet notochord, unlike the vertebrate spine, extends into the head. This gives the subphylum its name (*cephalo-* meaning 'relating to the head'). The nerve cord is only slightly larger in the head region than in the rest of the body, so that lancelets cannot be said to possess a true brain. Neither do they have any eyes, or other complex sense organs comparable to those of vertebrates.

Lancelets also have oral *cirri*, thin tentacle-like strands that hang in front of the mouth and act as sensory devices and as a filter for the water passing into the body. Water passes from the mouth into the large pharynx, which is lined by numerous gill-slits. The ventral surface of the pharynx contains a groove, called the endostyle, which, connected to a structure known as

Hatschek's pit, produces a film of mucus. Ciliary action pushes the mucus in a film over the surface of the gill slits, trapping suspended food particles as it does so. The mucus is collected in a second, dorsal, groove, and passed back to the rest of the digestive tract. Having passed through the gill slits, the water enters an atrium surrounding the pharynx, then exits the body via the *atriopore*.

The remainder of the digestive system consists of a simple tube running from the pharynx to the anus. A single blind-ending caecum branches off from the underside of the gut, with a lining able to phagocytize the food particles; a feature never found in vertebrates. It used to be thought that the caecum might be homologous to the liver of vertebrates, but this is now thought to be less likely.

Lancelets have no respiratory system, breathing solely through their skin, which consists of a simple epithelium. Despite the name, little if any respiration occurs in the gill slits, which are solely devoted to feeding. The circulatory system does resemble that of primitive fish in its general layout, but is much simpler, and does not include a heart. There are no blood cells, and no haemoglobin. The excretory system consists of segmented "kidneys" containing protonephridia instead of nephrons, and quite unlike those of vertebrates. Also unlike vertebrates, there are numerous, segmented gonads.

Taxonomy

The Cephalochordata is traditionally seen as a sister subphylum to the vertebrates, with which it is grouped together into a clade (sometimes called Notochordata) which in turn is the sister group to the simpler still Urochordata. Newer research suggests this may not be the case. The Cephalochordata may be the most basal subphylum of the chordates, while the sister group of the vertebrates may be the tunicates, previously known as the urochordates. However, other recent molecular studies (cit. in Benton 2005: 8) place cephalochordates nearer to vertebrates, and "most authors regard amphioxus as the closest relative of the Vertebrata on the basis of 10–15 [morphological] features that are not seen in tunicates".

The asymmetric nature of juveniles is unique to the cephalochordates and demonstrates (as do certain other features, including the seriated gonads) that lancelets are more derived than would be expected. This is a reminder that the "living fossil" representative of a basal clade has as long an evolutionary history as any other living thing, and thus is more derived than the actual primitive ancestor it otherwise so closely resembles. The following are the species recognised by ITIS. Other sources, for instance Tudge, show that there might be up to thirty species.

- Family Asymmetronidae
  - Genus *Asymmetron*
    - *Asymmetron lucayanum*
    - *Asymmetron maldivense*
  - Genus *Epigonichthys*
    - *Epigonichthys australis* (Raff, 1912)
    - *Epigonichthys bassanus* (Günther, 1884)
    - *Epigonichthys cingalense* (Kirkaldy, 1894)
    - *Epigonichthys cultellus* Peters, 1877
    - *Epigonichthys hectori* (Benham, 1901)
    - *Epigonichthys lucayanum* (Andrews, 1893)

   - *Epigonichthys maldivensis* (Foster Cooper, 1903)
- Family Branchiostomidae
  - o Genus *Branchiostoma*
    - *Branchiostoma belcheri*
    - *Branchiostoma californiense*
    - *Branchiostoma capense*
    - *Branchiostoma caribaeum*
    - *Branchiostoma clonaseum*
    - *Branchiostoma floridae*
    - *Branchiostoma lanceolatum*
    - *Branchiostoma minucauda*
    - *Branchiostoma moretonensis*
    - *Branchiostoma valdiviae*
    - *Branchiostoma virginiae.*

Hemichordata

Hemichordata is a phylum of marine deuterostome animals, generally considered the sister group of the echinoderms. They appear in the Lower or Middle Cambrian and include two main classes: Enteropneusta (acorn worms), and Pterobranchia. A third class, Planctosphaeroidea, is known only from the larva of a single species. The extinct class Graptolithina is closely related to the pterobranchs. Acorn worms are solitary worm-shaped organisms. They generally live in burrows and are deposit feeders, but some species are pharyngeal filter feeders. Pterobranchs are filter-feeders, mostly colonial, living in a collagenous tubular structure called a coenecium.

Structure

The body plan of hemichordates is characterized by a tripartite organisation. The anteroposterior axis is divided into three parts: the anterior prosome, the intermediate mesosome, and the posterior metasome.

The body of acorn worms is worm-shaped and divided into an anterior proboscis, an intermediate collar, and a posterior trunk. The proboscis is a muscular and ciliated organ used in locomotion and in the collection and transport of food particles. The mouth is located between the proboscis and the collar. The trunk is the longest part of the animal. It contains the pharynx, which is perforated with gill slits (or pharyngeal slits), the esophagus, a long intestine, and a terminal anus. It also contains the gonads.

The prosome of pterobranchs is specialised into a muscular and ciliated cephalic shield used in locomotion and in secreting the coenecium. The mesosome extends into one pair (in the genus *Rhabdopleura*) or several pairs (in the genus *Cephalodiscus*) of tentaculated arms used in filter feeding. The metasome, or trunk, contains a looped digestive tract, gonads, and extends into a contractile stalk that connects individuals to the other members of the colony, produced by asexual budding. In the genus *Cephalodiscus*, asexually produced individuals stay attached to the contractile stalk of the parent individual until completing their development. In the genus *Rhabdopleura*, zooids are permanently connected to the rest of the colony via a common stolon system.

They have a diverticulum of the foregut called a stomochord, previously thought to be related with the chordate notochord, but this is most likely the result of convergent evolution rather than homology. A hollow neural tube exists among some species (at least in early life), probably a primitive trait they share with the common ancestor of chordata and the rest of the deuterostomes.

Development

The hemichordates are the closest extant phylogenetic relatives of chordates among the invertebrates. Thus these marine worms, described to be the sister group of the echinoderms (such as sea urchins), are of great interest for the study of the origins of chordate development.

There are several species of hemichordates, with a moderate diversity of embryological development among these species. Hemichordates are classically known to develop in two ways, both directly and indirectly. Hemichordates are a phylum composed of two classes, the enteropneusts and the pterobranchs, both being forms of marine worm.

The enteropneusts have two developmental strategies: direct and indirect development. The indirect way of development is known to end in an extended pelagic plankotrophic tornaria larval stage, which means that this hemichordate exists in a larval stage that feeds on plankton before turning into an adult worm. Those species that are direct developing bypass this prolonged larval stage and develop directly into an adult worm.

The development of pterobranchs is studied only in *Rhabdopleura* from Plymouth, England and from Bermuda.

The following details the development of two popularly studied species of the hemichordata phylum *Saccoglossus kowalevskii* and *Ptychodera flava*. *Saccoglossus kowalevskii* is a direct developer and *Ptychodera flava* is an indirect developer. Most of what has been detailed in Hemichordate development has come from hemichordates that develop directly.

Ptychodera Flava

P. flava's early cleavage pattern is similar to that of *S. kowalevskii*. The first and second cleavages from the single cell zygote of *P. flava* are equal cleavages, are orthogonal to each other and both include the animal and vegetal poembryo has four blastomeres both in the vegetal and the animal pole. The fourth division occurs mainly in blastomeres in the animal pole, which divide transversally as well as equally to make eight blastomeres. The four vegetal blastomeres divide equatorially but unequally and they give rise to four big macromeres and four smaller micromeres. Once this fourth division has occurred the embryo has reached a 16 cell stage. *P. flava* has a 16 cell embryo with four vegetal micromeres, eight animal mesomeres and 4 larger macromeres. Further divisions occur until *P. flava* finishes the blastula stage and goes on to gastrulation. The animal mesomeres of *P. flava* go on to give rise to the larva's ectoderm, animal blastomeres also appear to give rise to these structures though the exact contribution varies from embryo to embryo.

The macromeres give rise to the posterior larval ectoderm and the vegetal micromeres give rise to the internal endomesodermal tissues. Studies done on the potential of the embryo at different stages have shown that at both the two and four cell stage of development *P. flava* blastomeres can go on to give rise to a tornaria larvae, so fates of these embryonic cells don't seem to be established till after this stage.

Saccoglossus Kowalevskii

Eggs of *S. kowalevskii* are oval in shape and become spherical in shape after fertilization. The first cleavage occurs from the animal to the vegetal pole and usually is equal though very often can also be unequal. The second cleavage to reach the embryos four cell stage also occurs from the animal to the vegetal pole in an approximately equal fashion though like the first cleavage it's possible to have an unequal division. The eight cell stage cleavage is latitudinal; so that each cell from the four cell stage goes on to make two cells. The fourth division occurs first in the cells of the animal pole which end up making 8 blastomeres (mesomeres) that are not radially symmetric, then the four vegetal pole blastomeres divide to make a level of four large blastomeres (macromeres) and four very small blastomeres (micromeres). The fifth cleavage occurs first in the animal cells and then in the vegetal cells to give a 32 cell blastomere. The sixth cleavage occurs in a similar order and completes a 64 cell stage, finally the seventh cleavage marks the end of the cleavage stage with a blastula with 128 blastomeres. This structure goes on to go thru gastrulation movements which will determine the body plan of the resulting gill slit larva, this larva will ultimately give rise to the marine acorn worm.

Genetic Control of Dorsal-Ventral Hemichordate Patterning

Much of the genetic work done on hemichordates has been done to make comparison with chordates, so it is obvious that many of the genetic markers identified in this group are also found in chordates or are homologous to chordates in some way. Studies of this nature have been done particularly on *S. kowalevskii*, and like chordates *S. kowalevskii* has dorsalizing bmp-like factors such as *bmp 2/4* which is homologous to Drosophila's decapentaplegic dpp. The expression of *bmp2/4* begins at the onset of gastrulation on the ectodermal side of the embryo, and as grastulation progresses its expression is narrowed down to the dorsal midline but is not expressed in the post anal tail. The bmp antagonist chordin is also expressed in the endoderm of gastrulating *S. kowalevskii*.

Besides these well known dorsalizing factors, further molecules known to be involved in dorsal ventral patterning are also present in *S. kowalevskii*, such as a netrin that groups with netrin gene class 1 and 2. Netrin is important in patterning of the neural system in chordates, as well as is the molecule Shh, but *S. kowalevskii* was only found to have one hh gene and it appears to be expressed in a region that is uncommon to where it is usually expressed in developing chordates along the ventral midline.

Classification

Hemichordata are divided into two classes: the Enteropneusta, commonly called acorn worms, and the Pterobranchia, which may include the graptolites. A third class, Planctosphaeroidea, is proposed based on a single species known only from larvae. The phylum contains about 120 living species. Hemichordata appears to be sister to the Echinodermata as Ambulacraria; Xenoturbellida may be basal to that grouping. Pterobranchia may be derived from within Enteropneusta, making Enteropneusta paraphyletic.

Echinoderm

Echinoderms (Phylum Echinodermata) are a phylum of marine animals. The adults are recognised easily by their (usually five-point) radial symmetry, and include such well-known animals as starfish, sea urchins, sand dollars, and sea cucumbers. Echinoderms are found at every ocean depth, from the intertidal zone to the abyssal zone.

The phylum contains about 7000 living species, making it the second-largest grouping of deuterostomes (a superphylum), after the chordates (which include the vertebrates, such as humans, sharks and frogs). Echinoderms are also the largest phylum that has no freshwater or terrestrial (land-based) representatives.

Aside from the hard-to-classify *Arkarua* (a Precambrian animal with Echinoderm-like pentamerous radial symmetry), the first definitive members of the phylum appeared near the start of the Cambrian period. The word "echinoderm" is made up from Greek *÷éíüäåñìá (echinóderma)*, "spiny skin", cf. *÷Ôíïò (echínos)*, "hedgehog; sea-urchin" and *äÝñìá (dérma)*, "skin", *echinodérmata* being the Greek plural form. The echinoderms are important both biologically and geologically. Biologically, there are few other groupings so abundant in the biotic desert of the deep sea, as well as shallower oceans. The more notably distinct trait, which most echinoderms have, is their remarkable powers of regeneration of tissue, organs, limbs, and of asexual reproduction, and in some cases, complete regeneration from a single limb. Geologically, the value of echinoderms is in their ossified skeletons, which are major contributors to many limestone formations, and can provide valuable clues as to the geological environment. Further, it is held by some scientists that the radiation of echinoderms was responsible for the Mesozoic revolution of marine life.

Taxonomy

Two main subdivisions of echinoderms are traditionally recognised: the more familiar motile Eleutherozoa, which encompasses the Asteroidea (starfish), Ophiuroidea (brittle stars), Echinoidea (sea urchins and sand dollars), and Holothuroidea (sea cucumbers); and the sessile Pelmatozoa, which consists of the crinoids and of the extinct blastoids and Paracrinoids. Some crinoids, however, namely the feather stars, are also highly motile (able to move themselves). A fifth class of Eleutherozoa consisting of just three species, the Concentricycloidea (sea daisies), were recently merged into the Asteroidea. The fossil record contains a host of other classes which do not appear to fall into any extant crown group.

Anatomy and Physiology

Echinoderms evolved from animals with bilateral symmetry. Although adult echinoderms possess pentaradial, or five-sided, symmetry, echinoderm larvae are ciliated, free-swimming organisms that organise in bilateral symmetry which makes them look like embryonic chordates. Later, the left side of the body grows at the expense of the right side, which is eventually absorbed. The left side then grows in a pentaradially symmetric fashion, in which the body is arranged in five parts around a central axis. All echinoderms exhibit fivefold radial symmetry in portions of their body at some stage of life, even if they have secondary bilateral symmetry. Many crinoids and some seastars exhibit symmetry in multiples of the basic five, with seastars such as *Helicoilaster* known to possess up to 50 arms, and the sea-lily *Comanthina schlegelii* boasting 200.

Skin and Skeleton

Echinoderms have a mesodermal skeleton composed of calcareous plates or ossicles. Despite the robustness of the individual skeletal modules, complete echinoderm skeletons are rare in the fossil record. This is because they quickly disarticulate (disconnect from each other) once the encompassing skin rots away, and in the absence of tissue there is nothing to hold the plates together. The modular construction is a result of the growth system employed by echinoderms, which adds new segments at the centre of the radial limbs, pushing the existing plates outwards, as if they are being "stacked". The spines of sea urchins are most readily lost, as each spine can be moved individually and is only loosely attached in life. A walk above a rocky shore will often reveal a large number of spineless but otherwise complete sea urchin skeletons.

Skeletal elements are also deployed in some specialised ways, such as the "Aristotle's lantern" of sea urchins, crinoids' stalks, and the supportive "lime ring" of sea cucumbers.

The epidermis (skin) itself consists of cells responsible for the support and maintenance of the skeleton, as well as pigment cells, mechanoreceptor cells (which detect motion on the animal's surface), and sometimes gland cells which secrete sticky fluids or even toxins.

The varied and often vivid colours of echinoderms are produced by the action of skin pigment cells. These may be light sensitive, and as a result many species change appearance completely as night falls. The reaction can happen quickly — the sea urchin *Centrostephanus longispinus* changes from jet black to grey-brown in just 50 minutes when exposed to light. The colours are produced by a variable combination of coloured pigments, such as the dark melanin, red carotinoids, and carotin proteins, which can be blue, green, or violet.

Water Vascular System

The water vascular system is a hydraulic system used by echinoderms, such as sea stars and sea urchins, for locomotion, food and waste transportation, and respiration. The system is composed of canals connecting numerous tube feet. Echinoderms move by alternately contracting muscles that force water into the tube feet, causing them to extend and push against the ground, then relaxing to allow the feet to retract. The exact structure of the system varies somewhat between the six classes of echinoderm.

Sea Stars

In sea stars, water enters the system through a sieve-like structure on the upper surface of the animal, called the madreporite. This overlies a small sac, or ampulla connected to a duct termed the stone canal, which is, as its name implies, commonly lined with calcareous material. The stone canal runs to a circular ring canal, from which radial canals run outwards along the ambulacral grooves. Each arm of a sea star has one such groove on its underside, while, in sea urchins, they run along the outside of the body.

Each side of the radial canals gives rise to a row of bulb-like ampullae, which are connected via lateral canals. In sea stars these are always staggered, so that an ampulla on the left follows one on the right, and so on down the length of the radial canal. The ampullae are connected to suckerlike podia, the entire structure is called a tube foot.

In most cases, the small lateral canals connecting the ampullae to the radial canal are of equal length, so that the tube feet are arranged in two rows, one along each side of the groove. In some species, however, there are alternately long and short lateral canals, giving the appearance of two rows on each side of the groove, for four in total. Contraction of the ampullae causes the podia to stretch as water is brought into them. This whole process allows for movement, and is quite powerful but extremely slow.

The central ring canal, in addition to connecting the radial canals to each other and to the stone canal, also has a number of other specialised structures on the inner surface. In between each radial canal, in many sea star species, there lies a muscular sac called a polian vesicle. The radial canal also has four or five pairs of complex pouches, called Tiedemann's bodies. These apparently produce coelomocytes, amoeboid cells somewhat similar to the blood cells of vertebrates.

Although the contents of the water vascular system are essentially sea water, apart from coelomocytes, the fluid also contains some protein and high levels of potassium salts.

Ophiuroids

Ophiuroids, the group including brittle stars and basket stars, have a somewhat different water vascular system from sea stars, despite their superficially similar appearance. The madreporite is located on the underside of the animal, usually in one of the jaw plates. The stone canal runs upwards to the ring canal, typically located in a circular depression on the upper (i.e. internal) surface of the jaws. The ring canal has four polian vesicles.

Ophiuroids have no ambulacral groove, and the radial canals instead run through the solid bone-like ossicles of the arms. Unlike sea stars, the tube feet are paired instead of staggered, and there are no ampullae. Instead, a simple valve at the upper end of the foot helps to control water pressure in the tube feet, along with contraction of the associated canals.

Sea urchins

The madreporite of sea urchins is located within one of the plates surrounding the anus on the upper surface of the animal. The stone canal descends from the madreporite to the ring canal, which lies around the oesophagus, and includes a number of polian vesicles. Because sea urchins have no arms, the five radial canals simply run along the inside of the solid skeletal "test", arching upwards towards the anus. The ampullae branching off from either side of the radial canals give rise to ten rows of tube feet, which penetrate through holes in the test to the outside. As in sea stars, the ampullae are arranged alternately, but in most (though not all) cases they split into two as they pass through the test before merging again on the outer side. The tube feet of sea urchins are often highly modified for different purposes. The radial canal ends in a small water-filled tentacle which protrudes through the uppermost plate of the ambulacral region.

Crinoids

Uniquely among echinoderms, crinoids have no madreporite. Instead, the oral surface is dotted within numerous minute ciliated funnels that run into the main body cavity. The ring canal has several small stone canals, located between the arms of the animal, but these open into the body cavity, and thus are only indirectly connected to the outside. The five radial canals run into the arms and branch several times to supply all of the individual branches and pinnules lining the arms. As in other echinoderms, the radial canals give rise to lateral canals, but there are no ampullae, and clusters of three tube feet branch from the ends of each canal, except around the mouth, where they are found singly. In the absence of ampullae, water pressure is maintained by the ring canal, which is surrounded by contractile muscle fibres.

Sea Cucumbers

The water vascular system of sea cucumbers has no connection to the outside, and is thus filled with the internal coelomic fluid, rather than sea water. The madreporite is present, but lies within the body cavity, just below the pharynx. The stone canal is relatively short. The ring canal normally has one to four polian vesicles, but in the order Apodida, there may be as many as fifty. The radial canals run through notches in the calcareous plates surrounding the mouth and then run along the ambulacral areas along the length of the body. Lateral canals run to both the tube feet and the large oral tentacles, all of which possess ampullae. The Apodida, which have no tube feet, also have no radial canals, with the canals to the tentacles branching off directly from the ring canal.

Other Organs

Although echinoderms possess a complete digestive gut, it is very simple, often simply leading directly from mouth to anus. It can generally be divided into a pharynx, stomach, intestine and anus or cloaca. Echinoderms also have a haemal system, and often also a *perihaemal system*. Both are derived from the coelom, and form an open and reduced circulatory system. This usually consists of a central ring and five radial vessels, although there is no true heart, and the blood often lacks any respiratory pigment. Gaseous exchange occurs by *dermal branchae* or *papulae* in seastars, *peristominal gills* in sea urchins, *genitial bursae* in brittle stars and *cloacal trees* in holothurians. Exchange of gases also takes place through tube feet. Echinoderms lack specialised excretory (waste disposal) organs and so nitrogenous waste, chiefly in the form of ammonia diffuses out through the respiratory surfaces.

They have a simple radial nervous system that consists of a modified nerve net — interconnected neurons with no central brain (although some do possess ganglia). Nerves radiate from central rings around the mouth into each arm or along the body; the branches of these nerves coordinate the movements of the organism. The gonads occupy the entire body cavities of sea urchins and sea cucumbers, while the less voluminous crinoids, brittle stars, and seastars have two gonads per arm. While the primitive condition is considered to be one genital aperture, many organisms have multiple holes through which eggs or sperm may be released.

Regeneration

Many echinoderms have remarkable powers of regeneration. Many species routinely autotomize and regenerate arms and viscera. Sea cucumbers often discharge parts of their internal organs if they perceive danger. The discharged organs and tissues are quickly regenerated. Sea urchins are constantly replacing spines lost through damage. Sea stars (asterozoa) and Sea lillys (crinozoa) readily lose and regenerate their arms. In most cases single severed arms cannot regenerate a complete individual in the absence of at least part of the disc.

However, in a few species a single arm can survive and develop into a complete individual. Some of these actively break off their arms for the purpose of asexual reproduction. During periods when they have lost the digestive tract, they live off stored nutrients and absorb dissolved organic matter directly from the water. The regeneration of lost parts involves both epimorphosis and morphallaxis. In epimorphosis stem cells - either from a reserve pool or those produced by dedifferentiation- form a blastema and generate new tissues. Morphallactic regeneration involves the movement and remodelling of existing tissues to replace lost parts. Direct transdifferentiation of one type of tissue to another during tissue replacement is also observed. The robust larval regeneration is responsible for many of them being popular model organisms in developmental biology.

Reproduction

Sexual Reproduction

Echinoderms become sexually mature after approximately two to three years, depending on the species and the environmental conditions. The eggs and sperm cells are released into open water, where fertilization takes place. The release of sperm and eggs is coordinated temporally in some species, and spatially in others. Internal fertilization has currently been observed in three species of sea star, three brittle stars and a deep water sea cucumber.

In some species of feather star, the embryos develop in special breeding bags, where the eggs are held until sperm released by a male happen to find them and fertilize the contents. This can also be found among sea urchins and sea cucumbers, where exhibit care for their young can occur, for instance in a few species of sand dollars who carry their young between the pricks of their oral side, and heart urchins possess breeding chambers. With brittle stars, special chambers can be developed near the stomach bags, in which the development of the young takes place. Species of sea cucumbers with specialised care for their offspring may also nurse the young in body cavities or on their surfaces. In rare cases, direct development without passing through a bilateral larval stage can occur in some sea stars and brittle stars. Another strategy that has evolved in some sea stars and brittle stars is the ability to reproduce asexually by dividing in two halves while they are small juveniles, while turning to sexual reproduction when they have reached sexual maturity.

Asexual Reproduction

One species of seastar reproduces asexually by parthenogenesis. In certain other asterozoans the adult organisms reproduce asexually for a while before they mature and reproduce sexually. In most of these species, they reproduce by transverse fission- with the disc splitting in two. Regrowth of both the disc and the arms occur giving an animal with some large arms and some small arms during the period of growth.

Though in most species at least part of the disc is needed for complete regeneration, in a few species of sea stars a single severed arm can grow into a complete individual over a period of several months. In at least some of these species, they actively use this as a method of asexual reproduction. A fracture develops on the lower surface of the arm and the arm pulls itself free from the body which holds onto the substrate during the process. During the period of regrowth, they have a few tiny arms and one large arm earning them the name of "comet forms". Asexual reproduction by fission has also been observed in adult holothuroidea (Sea cucumbers). They divide into two at a point closer to the anterior end from the middle. The two parts regenerate the missing organs over period of a few months.

The larvae of some echinoderm species are capable of asexual reproduction. These species belong to four of the major classes of echinoderms except crinozoans (as of 2011). Asexual reproduction in the planktonic larvae occurs through numerous modes.

They may autotomise parts that develop into secondary larvae, grow buds or undergo paratomy. The parts that are autotomised or the buds may develop directly into fully formed larvae or may develop through a gastrula or even a blastula stage. The parts that develop into the new larvae vary from the preoral hood (a mound like structure above the mouth), the side body wall, the postero-lateral arms or their rear ends.

The process of cloning costs the larva both in resources as well as in development time. They have been observed to undergo this process when food is plentiful or temperature conditions are right. It has also been proposed that cloning may occur to make use of the tissues that are normally lost in metamorphosis. Recent research has shown that the larvae of some sand dollars clone themselves when they detect predators (by sensing dissolved fish mucus). Asexual reproduction produces many smaller larvae that escape planktivorous fish better.

Larval Development

The development of an echinoderm begins with a bilaterally symmetrical embryo, with a coeloblastula developing first. Gastrulation marks the opening of the "second mouth" that places them within the deuterostomes, and the mesoderm, which will host the skeleton, migrates inwards. The secondary body cavity, the coelom, forms by the partitioning of three body cavities. Upon metamorphosis, each taxon produces a distinct planktonic larva, which varies in shape among the classes. Larval stages with prominent "arms" are often referred to as pluteus larvae (often with a prefix to denote taxon). The left hand side of the larva develops into the adult organism while the right hand side eventually being absorbed; the left hand side typically becomes the oral plate.

Distribution and Habitat

Echinoderms are globally distributed in almost all depths, latitudes and environments in the ocean. They reach highest diversity in reef environments but are also widespread on shallow shores, around the poles — refugia where crinoids are at their most abundant — and throughout the deep ocean, where bottom-dwelling and burrowing sea cucumbers are common — sometimes accounting for up to 90% of organisms. While almost all echinoderms are benthic — that is, they live on the sea floor — some sea-lilies can swim at great velocity for brief periods of time, and a few deep-sea sea cucumbers are fully floating. Some crinoids are pseudo-planktonic, attaching themselves to floating logs and debris, although this behaviour was exercised most extensively in the Paleozoic, before competition from such organisms as barnacles restricted the extent of the behaviour. Some sea cucumbers employ a similar strategy, hitching lifts by attaching to the sides of fish. The larvæ of echinoderms, especially starfish and sea urchins, are pelagic, and with the aid of ocean currents can swim great distances, reinforcing the global distribution of the phylum.

Mode of Life

Feeding: The modes of feeding vary greatly between the constituent taxa. Crinoids and some brittle stars tend to be passive filter-feeders, absorbing suspended particles from passing water; sea urchins are grazers, sea cucumbers deposit feeders, and seastars are active hunters. Crinoids employ a large net-like structure to sieve water as it is swept by currents, and to absorb any particles of matter sinking from the ocean overhead. Once a particle touches the arms of the creature, the tube feet act to swish it to the central mouth of the crinoid, where it is ingested, nutrients removed, and the remains egested through its anus to the underlying water column.

Many sea urchins graze on the surfaces of rocks, scraping off the thin layer of algae covering the surfaces. Other toothless breeds devour smaller organisms, which they may catch with their tube feet, whole. Sand dollars may perform suspension feeding. Sea cucumbers may be suspension feeders, sucking vast quantities of sea water through their guts and absorbing any useful matter. Others use their feeding apparatus to actively capture food from the sea floor. Yet others deploy their feeding apparatus as a net, in which smaller organisms become ensnared.

While some sea stars are detritovores, extracting the organic material from mud, and others mimic the crinoids' filter feeding, most are active hunters, attacking other sea stars or shellfish. The latter are seized and held by the tube feet; sea stars then stiffen their legs, expanding the shell. The sea stars can use connective tissue to lock their arms in place and maintain a force on the prey while exerting minimal effort; the unfortunate victim must expend energy resisting the force with its adductor muscle. When the adductor tires, the sea star can insert its stomach through the opening and release gastric juices, digesting the prey alive.

Avoiding Predation

Despite their low nutrition value and the abundance of indigestible calcite, echinoderms are the prey of many organisms, such as crabs, sharks, sea birds and larger starfish. Defensive strategies employed include the presence of spines, toxins, which can be inherent or delivered through the tube feet, and the discharge of sticky entangling threads by sea cucumbers. Being stabbed by a sea urchin may result in painful injury.

Ecology

Echinoderms provide a key ecological role in ecosystems. For example, the grazing of sea urchins reduces the rate of colonization of bare rock; the burrowing of sand dollars and sea cucumbers depleted the sea floor of nutrients and encouraged deeper penetration of the sea floor, increasing the depth to which oxygenation occurs and allowing a more complex ecological tiering to develop. Starfish and brittle stars prevent the growth of algal mats on coral reefs, which would obstruct the filter-feeding constituent organisms. Some sea urchins can bore into solid rock; this bioerosion can destabilise rock faces and release nutrients into the ocean. It has also been estimated that they capture and sequester about 0.1 gigatonnes of carbon per year as calcium carbonate, making them important contributors in the global carbon cycle.

The echinoderms are also the staple diet of many organisms, most notably the otter; conversely, many sea cucumbers provide a habitat for parasites, including crabs, worms and snails. The extinction of large quantities of echinoderms appears to have caused a subsequent overrunning of ecosystems by seaweed, or the destruction of an entire reef.

Evolution

The first universally accepted echinoderms appear in the Lower Cambrian period (Paul and Smith 1984). Echinoderms left behind an extensive fossil record. Despite this, there are numerous conflicting hypotheses on their phylogeny. Based on their bilateral larvae, many zoologists argue that echinoderm ancestors were bilateral and that their coelom had three pairs of spaces (trimeric).

Some have proposed that radial symmetry arose in a free-moving echinoderm ancestor and that sessile groups were derived several times independently from free-moving ancestors. Unfortunately, this view does not address the significance of radial symmetry as an adaptation for a sessile existence.

The more traditional view is that the first echinoderms were sessile, became radial as an adaptation to that existence, and then gave rise to free-moving groups. This view perceives the evolution of endoskeletal plates with stereom structure and of external ciliary grooves for feeding as early echinoderm developments. The extinct members of paraphyletic Homalozoa, commonly referred to as carpoids, had stereom ossicles but were not radially symmetrical, and the status of their water-vascular system is not known. Further, extinct members of the Class Helicoplacoidea possessed three, true ambulacral grooves, and their mouth was on the side of their body. Attachment to a substratum would have selected for radial symmetry and may have marked the origin of the Class Crinoidea. Members of Crinoidea, along with the extinct members of Class Cystoidea, were primitively attached to a substratum by an aboral stalk.

An ancestor that became free-moving might have given rise to Asteroidea, Ophiuroidia, Holothuroidea, and Echinoidea.

Use by Humans

Echinoderms sometimes pose a health threat to humans. The fine structure of the spines of certain species of sea urchins means that if the spine pierces the flesh, it may break off when an attempt is made to remove it. It may require patience — or the assistance of a physician — to fully remove the remaining piece of spine. In 2010, 373,000 tonnes of echinoderms were harvested, mainly for consumption. These were mainly sea cucumbers (158,000 tonnes) and sea urchins (73,000 tonnes).

Sea cucumbers are considered a delicacy in some countries of south east Asia; particularly popular are the (Pineapple) roller *Thelenota ananas* (*susuhan*) and the red *Halodeima edulis*. They are well known as *bêche de mer* or *Trepang* in China and Indonesia. The sea cucumbers are dried, and the potentially poisonous entrails removed. The strong poisons of the sea cucumbers are often psychoactive, but their effects are not well studied. It does appear that some sea cucumber toxins restrain the growth rate of tumour cells, which has sparked interest from cancer researchers. The gonads of sea urchins are consumed particularly in Japan, Peru, Spain and France. The taste is described as soft and melting, like a mix of seafood and fruit. The quality depends on the colour, which can range from light yellow to bright orange. The calcareous tests or shells of echinoderms are used as a source of lime by farmers in areas where limestone is unavailable; indeed, 4,000 tons of the animals are used annually for this purpose. This trade is often carried out in conjunction with shellfish farmers, for whom the starfish pose a major irritation by eating their stocks. Sea-urchin and sand dollar skeletons are popular collectibles, as are dried starfish.

Origins

The majority of animals more complex than jellyfish and other Cnidarians are split into two groups, the protostomes and deuterostomes, and chordates are deuterostomes. It seems very likely the 555 million-year-old *Kimberella* was a member of the protostomes. If so, this means the protostome and deuterostome lineages must have split some time before *Kimberella* appeared

— at least 558 million years ago, and hence well before the start of the Cambrian 541 million years ago. The Ediacaran fossil *Ernietta*, from about 549 to 543 million years ago, may represent a deuterostome animal.

Fossils of one major deuterostome group, the echinoderms (whose modern members include starfish, sea urchins and crinoids), are quite common from the start of the Cambrian, 542 million years ago. The Mid Cambrian fossil *Rhabdotubus johanssoni* has been interpreted as a pterobranch hemichordate. Opinions differ about whether the Chengjiang fauna fossil *Yunnanozoon*, from the earlier Cambrian, was a hemichordate or chordate.

Another fossil, *Haikouella lanceolata*, also from the Chengjiang fauna, is interpreted as a chordate and possibly a craniate, as it shows signs of a heart, arteries, gill filaments, a tail, a neural chord with a brain at the front end, and possibly eyes — although it also had short tentacles round its mouth. *Haikouichthys* and *Myllokunmingia*, also from the Chengjiang fauna, are regarded as fish. *Pikaia*, discovered much earlier but from the Mid Cambrian Burgess Shale, is also regarded as a primitive chordate. On the other hand fossils of early chordates are very rare, since non-vertebrate chordates have no bones or teeth, and only one has been reported for the rest of the Cambrian.The evolutionary relationships between the chordate groups and between chordates as a whole and their closest deuterostome relatives have been debated since 1890.

Studies based on anatomical, embryological, and paleontological data have produced different "family trees". Some closely linked chordates and hemichordates, but that idea is now rejected. Combining such analyses with data from a small set of ribosome RNA genes eliminated some older ideas, but open the possibility that tunicates (urochordates) are "basal deuterostomes", surviving members of the group from which echinoderms, hemichordates and chordates evolved. Some researchers believe that, within the chordates, craniates are most closely related to cephalochordates, but there are also reasons for regarding tunicates (urochordates) as craniates' closest relatives. One other phylum, Xenoturbellida, appears to be basal within the deuterostomes, closer to the original deuterostomes than to the chordates, echinoderms and hemichordates. Since chordates have left a poor fossil record, attempts have been made to calculate the key dates in their evolution by molecular phylogenetics techniques - by analyzing biochemical differences, mainly in RNA. One such study suggested deuterostomes arose before 900 million years ago and the earliest chordates around 896 million years ago. However, molecular estimates of dates often disagree with each other and with the fossil record, and their assumption that the molecular clock runs at a known constant rate has been challenged.

Classification

Taxonomy: The following schema is from the third edition of *Vertebrate Palaeontology*. The invertebrate chordate classes are from Fishes of the World. While it is structured so as to reflect evolutionary relationships (similar to a cladogram), it also retains the traditional ranks used in Linnaean taxonomy.

- Phylum Chordata
  - Subphylum Tunicata (Urochordata) — (tunicates; 3,000 species)
    - Class Ascidiacea (sea squirts)
    - Class Thaliacea (salps)
    - Class Appendicularia (larvaceans)
    - Class Sorberacea
  - Subphylum Cephalochordata (Acraniata) — (lancelets; 30 species)
    - Class Leptocardii (lancelets)
  - Subphylum Vertebrata (Craniata) (vertebrates — animals with backbones; 57,674 species)
    - Infraphylum incertae sedis
    - Superclass 'Agnatha' paraphyletic (jawless vertebrates; 100+ species)
    - Class Myxini (hagfish; 65 species)
    - Class Petromyzontida (lampreys)
    - Class †Conodonta
    - Infraphylum Gnathostomata (jawed vertebrates)

- Superclass incertae sedis
- Class †Placodermi (Paleozoic armoured forms)
- Class Chondrichthyes (cartilaginous fish; 900+ species)
- Class †Acanthodii (Paleozoic "spiny sharks")
- Superclass Osteichthyes (bony fish; 30,000+ species)
- Class Actinopterygii (ray-finned fish; about 30,000 species)
- Class Sarcopterygii (lobe-finned fish: 8 species)
- Superclass Tetrapoda (four-limbed vertebrates; 28,000+ species)
- Class Amphibia (amphibians; 6,000 species)
- Class Reptilia (reptiles; 9,000+ species)
- Class †Synapsida (synapsids; 4,000+ species)
- Class Aves (birds; 8,800–10,000 species)
- Class Mammalia (mammals; 5,700+ species).

Chapter 4

Vertebrates and Invertebrates

Invertebrate

Invertebrates are animal species that do not develop a vertebral column. This in effect includes all animals apart from the subphylum Vertebrata. Familiar examples of invertebrates include insects, snails, and starfish. Taxonomically speaking "invertebrate" is no more than a term of convenience; only about 3% of animal species include a vertebral column in their anatomy.

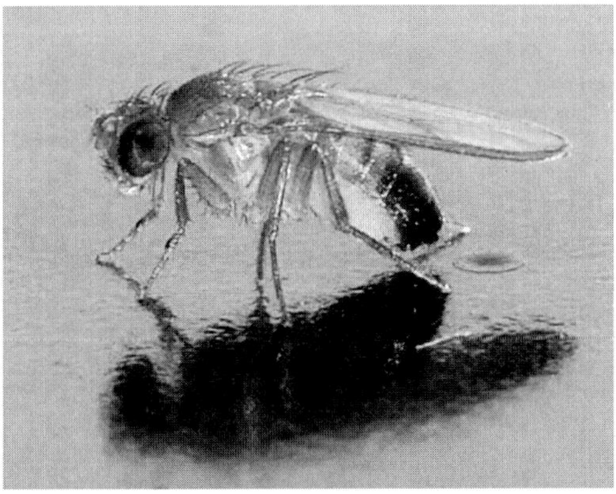

Figure: The common fruit fly, Drosophila melanogaster, has been the subject of much research

In other words all animals except those in the chordate subphylum Vertebrata (fish, amphibians, reptiles, birds, and mammals) are regarded as invertebrates. What is more, many an individual invertebrate taxon has a greater number and variety of species than the entire subphylum Vertebrata, In fact some of the so-called invertebrata, such as the Chaetognatha and Hemichordata, are more closely related the Chordata than to other invertebrate phyla. Invertebrates form a massively paraphyletic group.

It is generally accepted that the phyla comprising modern Eukaryota share a common multicellular ancestor, but with the sole exception of one subphylum of the phylum Chordata, all those phyla are classed as invertebrates along with two of the three subphyla in the Chordata: Tunicata and Cephalochordata. These two, plus all the other known invertebrates, have only one cluster of Hox genes, while the vertebrates have duplicated their original cluster more than once. Within palaeozoology and palaeobiology, invertebrates are often studied within the fossil discipline called invertebrate palaeontology.

Etymology

The word *invertebrate* comes from the word *vertebrate*, with the prefix *in-* attached to it. Thus, the word indicates that which lacks vertebrae.

Taxonomic Significance

The term Invertebrate promotes a great deal of confusion among non-biologists. It does not refer to any particular taxon in the same way that Arthropoda, Vertebrata or Manidae would do. Each of those examples describes a presumably monophyletically valid taxon, say a phylum, subphylum or family. In referring to taxonomy of the Animalia, "invertebrata" is a term of convenience, not a taxon; it has very little circumscriptional significance except arguably within the Chordata.

The Vertebrata as a subphylum comprises such a small proportion of the Metazoa that to speak of the kingdom Animalia in terms of "Vertebrata" and "Invertebrata" would be about as practical as classifying animals into mayflies and non-mayflies, or transport into rowing boats and non-rowing boats.

It would be logically correct to do so, and rowing boats as such do form a practical group, but speaking of "non-rowing boats" would lump together land, sea, air and space transport in ways that rarely would be useful. In formal taxonomy of the Animalia there are higher level attributes that logically should precede the presence or absence of the vertebral column in constructing a cladogram, for example, the presence of a notochord. That would at least circumscribe the Chordata. However, even the notochord would be a less fundamental criterion than aspects of embryological development and symmetry or perhaps bauplan. The resultant cladistic structure would not resemble anything like a binary split into vertebrates and invertebrates. At the same time, there certainly is no reason to avoid the use of the terms Invertebrata or invertebrates when they are convenient, but it is important not to confuse the terms with the names or relationships of actual taxa.

Characteristics

The trait that is common to all invertebrates is the absence of a vertebral column: this creates a distinction between invertebrates and vertebrates. Being animals, invertebrates are heterotrophs, and require sustenance in the form of the consumption of other organisms. With a few exceptions, such as the Porifera, invertebrates generally have bodies composed of differentiated tissues. There is also typically a digestive chamber with one or two openings to the exterior. Like vertebrates, most invertebrates reproduce at least partly through sexual reproduction. They produce specialised reproductive cells that undergo meiosis to produce smaller, motile spermatozoa or larger, non-motile ova. These fuse to form zygotes, which develop into new individuals. Others are capable of asexual reproduction, or sometimes, both methods of reproduction.

Phyla

The term invertebrate covers several phyla. One of these are the sponges (Porifera). They were long thought to have diverged from other animals early. They lack the complex organisation found in most other phyla. Their cells are differentiated, but in most cases not organised into distinct tissues. Sponges typically feed by drawing in water through pores. Some speculate that sponges are not so primitive, but may instead be secondarily simplified. The Ctenophora and the Cnidaria, which includes sea anemones, corals, and jellyfish, are radially symmetric and have digestive chambers with a single opening, which serves as both the mouth and the anus. Both have distinct tissues, but they are not organised into organs. There are only two main germ layers, the ectoderm and endoderm, with only scattered cells between them. As such, they are sometimes called diploblastic. The Echinodermata are radially symmetric and exclusively marine, including starfish (Asteroidea), sea urchins, (Echinoidea), brittle stars (Ophiuroidea), sea cucumbers (Holothuroidea) and feather stars (Crinoidea).

Other phyla of invertebrates are the Hemichordata, or acorn worms, and the Chaetognatha, or arrow worms. The largest animal phylum is also included within invertebrates: the Arthropoda, including insects, spiders, crabs, and their kin. All these organisms have a body divided into repeating segments, typically with paired appendages. In addition, they possess a hardened exoskeleton that is periodically shed during growth. Two smaller phyla, the Onychophora and Tardigrada, are close relatives of the arthropods and share these traits. The Nematoda or roundworms, are perhaps the second largest animal phylum, and are also invertebrates. Roundworms are typically microscopic, and occur in nearly every environment where there is water. A number are important parasites. Smaller phyla related to them are the Kinorhyncha, Priapulida, and Loricifera. These groups have a reduced coelom, called a pseudocoelom. Other invertebrates include the Nemertea or ribbon worms, and the Sipuncula. Another phylum is Platyhelminthes, the flatworms. These were originally considered primitive, but it now appears they developed from more complex ancestors. Flatworms are acoelomates, lacking a body cavity, as are their closest relatives, the microscopic Gastrotricha. The Rotifera or rotifers, are common in aqueous environments. Invertbrates also include the Acanthocephala or spiny-headed worms, the Gnathostomulida, Micrognathozoa, and the Cycliophora.

Also included are two of the most successful animal phyla, the Mollusca and Annelida. The former, which is the second-largest animal phylum by number of described species, includes animals such as snails, clams, and squids, and the latter comprises the segmented worms, such as earthworms and leeches. These two groups have long been considered close relatives because of the common presence of trochophore larvae, but the annelids were considered closer to the arthropods because they are both segmented. Now, this is generally considered convergent evolution, owing to many morphological and genetic differences between the two phyla. Other phyla include Acoelomorpha, Brachiopoda, Bryozoa, Entoprocta, Phoronida, and Xenoturbellida.

History

Some of the first animal fossils appear to be those of invertebrates. 665-million-year-old fossils in the Trezona Formation at Trezona Bore, West Central Flinders, South Australia have been interpreted as being early sponges. Some paleontologists suggest that animals appeared much earlier, possibly as early as 1 billion years ago. Trace fossils such as tracks and burrows found in the Tonian era indicate the presence of triploblastic worms, like metazoans, roughly as large (about 5 mm wide) and complex as earthworms. Around 453 MYA, animals began diversifying, and many of the important groups of invertebrates diverged from one another. Fossils of invertebrates are found in various types of sediment from the Phanerozoic. Fossils of invertebrates are commonly used in stratigraphy.

Classification

Carl Linnaeus divided these animals into only two groups, the Insecta and the now-obsolete Vermes (worms). Jean-Baptiste Lamarck, who was appointed to the position of "Curator of Insecta and Vermes" at the Muséum National d'Histoire Naturelle in 1793, both coined the term "invertebrate" to describe such animals, and divided the original two groups into ten, by splitting Arachnida and Crustacea from the Linnean Insecta, and Mollusca, Annelida, Cirripedia, Radiata, Coelenterata and Infusoria from the Linnean Vermes. They are now classified into over 30 phyla, from simple organisms such as sea sponges and flatworms to complex animals such as arthropods and molluscs.

Significance of the Group

Invertebrates are animals *without* a vertebral column. This has led to the conclusion that *in*vertebrates are a group that deviates from the norm, vertebrates. This has been said to be due to the fact that researchers in the past, such as Lamarck, viewed vertebrates as a "standard": in Lamarck's theory of evolution, he believed that characteristics acquired through the evolutionary process involved not only survival, but also progression toward a "higher form", to which humans and vertebrates were closer than invertebrates were. Although goal-directed evolution has been abandoned, the distinction of invertebrates and vertebrates persists to this day, even though the grouping has been noted to be "hardly natural or even very sharp." Another reason cited for this continued distinction is that Lamarck created a precedent through his classifications which is now difficult to escape from. It's also possible that some humans believe that, they themselves being vertebrates, the group deserves more attention than invertebrates. In any event, in the 1968 edition of *Invertebrate Zoology*, it is noted that "division of the Animal Kingdom into vertebrates and invertebrates is artificial and reflects human bias in favour of man's own relatives." The book also points out that the group lumps a vast number of species together, so that no one characteristic describes all invertebrates. In addition, some species included are only remotely related to one another, with some more related to vertebrates than other invertebrates.

In Research

Two of the most commonly studied model organisms are invertebrates: the fruit fly *Drosophila melanogaster* and the nematode *Caenorhabditis elegans*. They have long been the most intensively studied model organisms, and were among the first life-forms to be genetically sequenced. This was facilitated by the severely reduced state of their genomes, but many genes, introns, and linkages have been lost. Analysis of the starlet sea anemone genome has emphasised the importance of sponges, placozoans, and choanoflagellates, also being sequenced, in explaining the arrival of 1500 ancestral genes unique to animals. Arthropods, especially insects, are often used by forensic scientists. For example, some invertebrates are attracted to dead bodies.

Protozoa

Protozoa are a diverse group of unicellular eukaryotic organisms, many of which are motile. Originally, protozoa had been defined as unicellular protists with animal-like behaviour, e.g., movement. Protozoa were regarded as the partner group of protists to protophyta, which have plant-like behaviour, e.g., photosynthesis.

Terminology

Following the Greek root of the name cillia, the singular form is *protozoon* /proŠtYÈzoŠ.Rn/. Its use has, however, partially been replaced by the word *protozoan*, which was originally only used as an adjective. In the same manner the plural form *protozoans* is sometimes being used instead of *protozoa*.

In general, protozoa are referred to as animal-like protists because of movement (motile). However, both protozoa and protists are paraphyletic groups (not including all genetic relatives of the group). For example, *Entamoeba* is more closely related to humans than to *Euglena*. "Protozoa" is considered an outdated classification in more formal contexts. However, the term is still used in children's education.

While there is no exact definition for the term *protozoa*, it often refers to a unicellular heterotrophic protist, such as the amoeba and ciliates. The term *algae* is used for microorganisms that photosynthesize.

However, distinction between protozoa and algae is often vague. For example, the algae *Dinobryon* has chloroplasts for photosynthesis, but it can also feed on organic matter and is motile. Protozoa is sometimes considered a subkingdom. It was traditionally considered a phylum under Animalia referring to unicellular animals, with Metazoa referring to multicellular animals.

Motility and Digestion

Tulodens are 2 of the slow-moving form of protozoa. They move around with whip-like tails called flagella, hair-like structures called cilia, or foot-like structures called pseudopodia. Others do not move at all. Protozoa may absorb food via their cell membranes, some, e.g., amoebas, surround food and engulf it, and yet others have openings or "mouth pores" into which they sweep food. All protozoa digest their food in stomach-like compartments called vacuoles.

Pellicle

The pellicle is a thin layer supporting the cell membrane in various protozoa, protecting them and allowing them to retain their shape, especially during locomotion, allowing the organism to be more hydrodynamic. They vary from flexible and elastic to rigid. Although somewhat stiff, the pellicle is also flexible and allows the protist to fit into tighter spaces. In ciliates and Apicomplexa, it is formed from closely packed vesicles called alveoli. In euglenids, it is formed from protein strips arranged spirally along the length of the body. Examples of protists with a pellicle are the euglenoids and the paramecium, a ciliate. The pellicle consists of many bacteria that adhere to the surface by their attachment pili. Thus, attachment pili allow the organisms to remain in the broth, from which they take nutrients, while they congregate near air, where the oxygen concentration is greatest.

Ecological Role

As components of the micro- and meiofauna, protozoa are an important food source for microinvertebrates. Thus, the ecological role of protozoa in the transfer of bacterial and algal production to successive trophic levels is important. As predators, they prey upon unicellular or filamentous algae, bacteria, and microfungi. Protozoa are both herbivores and consumers in the decomposer link of the food chain. They also control bacteria populations and biomass to some extent. Protozoa such as the malaria parasites (*Plasmodium* spp.), trypanosomes and leishmania, are also important as parasites and symbionts of multicellular animals.

Classification

Protozoa were previously often grouped in the kingdom of Protista, together with the plant-like algae and fungus-like slime molds. As a result of 21st-century systematics, protozoa, along with ciliates, mastigophorans, and apicomplexans, are arranged as animal-like protists. With the possible exception of Myxozoa, protozoa are not categorized as Metazoa. Protozoa are unicellular organisms and are often called the animal-like protists because they subsist entirely on other organisms for food. Most protozoa can move about on their own. Amoebas,

Paramecia, and Trypanosomes are all examples of animal-like Protists.

Sub-Groups

The classification of protozoa has been and remains a problematic area of taxonomy. Where they are available DNA sequences are used as the basis for classification but for the majority of described protozoa such material is not available. They have been and still are mostly on the basis of their morphology and for the parasitic species their hosts. Protozoa have been divided traditionally on the basis of their means of locomotion.

Flagellate

Flagellates are organisms with one or more whip-like organelles called flagella. Some cells in animals may be flagellate, for instance the spermatozoa of most phyla. Flowering plants do not produce flagellate cells, but ferns, mosses, green algae, some gymnosperms and other closely related plants do. Likewise, most fungi do not produce cells with flagellae, but the primitive fungal chytrids do. Many protists take the form of single-celled flagellates.The word *flagellate* describe a particular construction of eukaryotic organism and its means of motion. The term does not imply any specific relationship or classification of the organisms that possess flagellae. However, the term "flagellate" is included in other terms (such as "dinoflagellate" and "zooflagellate") which often are more formally characterised.

Form and Behaviour

Eukaryotic flagella are supported by microtubules in a characteristic arrangement, with nine fused pairs surrounding two central singlets. These arise from a basal body or kinetosome, with microtubule roots that are an important part of the cell's brain. In some, for instance, they support a cytostome or mouth, where food is ingested. The flagella often supports hairs, called mastigonemes, or contain rods. Their ultrastructure plays an important role in classifying eukaryotes. In protoctists and microscopic animals, flagella are generally used for propulsion. They may also be used to create a current that brings in food. In most things, one or more flagella are located at or near the anterior of the cell e.g. Euglena. Often there is one directed forwards and one trailing behind. Among animals, fungi, and Choanozoa, which make up a group called the opisthokonts, there is a single posterior flagellum. They are from the phylum Mastigophora. They can cause diseases and they can make their own food. They reproduce by binary fission.

Apicomplexa

The Apicomplexa (also referred to as Apicomplexia) are a large group of protists, most of which possess a unique organelle called apicoplast and an *apical complex* structure involved in penetrating a host's cell. They are unicellular, spore-forming, and exclusively parasites of animals. Motile structures such as flagella or pseudopods are present only in certain gamete stages. This is a diverse group including organisms such as coccidia, gregarines, piroplasms, haemogregarines, and plasmodia. Diseases caused by apicomplexan organisms include, but are not limited to:

- Babesiosis (*Babesia*)
- Malaria (*Plasmodium*)
- Coccidian diseases including:
    - Cryptosporidiosis (*Cryptosporidium parvum*)
    - Cyclosporiasis (*Cyclospora cayetanensis*)
    - Isosporiasis (*Isospora belli*)
    - Toxoplasmosis (*Toxoplasma gondii*)

The name of the taxon *Apicomplexa* is derived from two Latin words - *apex* (top) and *complexus* (infolds) - and refers to a set of organelles in the sporozoite. The older taxon Sporozoa grouped the *Apicomplexa* together with the Microsporidia and Myxosporida. This grouping is no longer regarded as biologically valid and its use is discouraged.

History

The first apicomplexan protozoan was seen by Antony van Leeuwenhoek who in 1674 saw oocysts of *Eimeria stiedae* in the gall bladder of a rabbit. The first member of the phylum to be named (by Dufour in 1828) was *Gregarina ovata* in earwigs. Since then many more have been identified and named. During the quarter century 1826-1850, 41 species and 6 genera of

Apicomplexa were named. In the quarter century 1951-1975, 1873 new species and 83 new genera were added.

Taxonomy

The field of classifying Apicomplexa is in flux and classification has changed throughout the years since it was formally named in 1970.

1987

By 1987 a comprehensive survey of the phylum was completed: in all, 4516 species and 339 genera had been named. They consisted of:

- the gregarines (subclass Gregarinasida) with 1624 named species and 231 named genera
- the hemogregarines (family Haemogregarinidae) with 399 species and 4 genera
- the eimeriorins (order Eimeriorida) with 1771 species and 43 genera
- the hemospororids (order Haemosporasina) with 444 species and 9 genera
- the piroplasmids (order Piroplasmorida) with 173 species and 20 genera
- and a few others (105 species and 32 genera)

Although there has been considerable revision of this phylum (the order Haemosporidia now has 17 genera rather than 9) it seems likely these numbers are still approximately correct.

Jacques Euzéby (1988)

Jacques Euzéby in 1988 created a new class Haemosporidiasina by merging subclass Piroplasmasina and suborder Haemospororina.

- Subclass Gregarinasina (the gregarines)
- Subclass Coccidiasina
    - Suborder Adeleorina (the adeleorins)
    - Suborder Eimeriorina (the eimeriorins)
- Subclass Haemosporidiasina
    - Order Chromatorida
    - Order Achromatorida

Roberts and Janovy (1996)

Roberts and Janovy in 1996 divided the phylum into the following subclasses and suborders (omitting classes and orders):

- Subclass Gregarinasina (the gregarines)
- Subclass Coccidiasina
  - o Suborder Adeleorina (the adeleorins)
  - o Suborder Eimeriorina (the eimeriorins)
  - o Suborder Haemospororina (the haemospororins)
- Subclass Piroplasmasina (the piroplasms)

These form the following five taxonomic groups:

1. The gregarines are generally one-host parasites of invertebrates.
2. The adeleorins are one-host parasites of invertebrates or vertebrates, or two-host parasites that alternately infect haematophagous (blood-feeding) invertebrates and the blood of vertebrates.
3. The eimeriorins are a diverse group that includes one host species of invertebrates, two-host species of invertebrates, one-host species of vertebrates and two-host species of vertebrates. The eimeriorins are frequently called the coccidia. Somewhat confusingly this term is often used to include the adeleorins.
4. Haemospororins often known as the malaria parasites, are two-host Apicomplexa that parasitize blood-feeding dipteran fies and the blood of various tetrapod vertebrates.
5. Piroplasms where all the species included are two-host parasites infecting ticks and vertebrates.

Perkins (2000)

This scheme is taken from Perkins et al. It is outdated as the Perkinsidae have since been recognised as a sister group to the dinoflagellates rather that the Apicomplexia. The remainder of the scheme appears to be valid:

- Class Aconoidasida: Conoid present only in the ookinete of some species

- Order Haemospororida: Macrogamete and microgamete develop separately. Syzygy does not occur. Ookinete has a conoid. Sporozoites have three walls. Heteroxenous : alternates between vertebrate host (in which merogony occurs) and invertebrate host (in which sporogony occurs). Usually blood parasites, transmitted by blood-sucking insects.
- Order Piroplasmorida
- Class Conoidasida
  - o Subclass Gregarinasina
    - — Order Archigregarinorida
    - — Order Eugregarinorida
    - — Suborder Adeleorina
    - — Suborder Eimeriorina
    - — Order Neogregarinorida
  - o Subclass Coccidiasina
    - — Order Agamococcidiorida
    - — Order Eucoccidiorida
    - — Order Ixorheorida
    - — Order Protococcidiorida
- Class Perkinsasida
- Order Perkinsorida
- Family Perkinsidae

General Morphological Features

All members of this phylum have an infectious stage - the sporozoite - which possess three distinct structures in an apical complex. The apical complex consists of a set of spirally arranged microtubules (the conoid), a secretory body (the rhoptry) and one or more polar rings. Additional slender electron dense secretory bodies (micronemes) surrounded by one or two polar rings may also be present. It is this structure that gives the phylum its name. A further group of spherical organelles are distributed throughout the cell rather than being localized at the apical complex and are known as the dense granules. These typically have a mean diametre of about 0.7 micrometres. Secretion of the dense-granule content takes place after parasite invasion and localization within the parasitophorous vacuole and persists for several minutes

Other morphological findings that are common to all members of this phylum include:

- The nucleus is haploid.
- Flagellae are found only in the motile gamete. These are posteriorly directed and vary in number (usually one to three).
- Basal bodies are present. Although hemosporidians and piroplasmids have normal triplets of microtubules in their basal bodies and coccidians and gregarines have 9 singlets.
- The mitochondria have tubular cristae.
- A Golgi apparatus is present.
- Centrioles, chloroplasts, ejectile organelles and inclusions are absent.
- Colourless plastids are present in some species.
- The cell is surrounded by a pellicle of three membrane layers (the alveolar structure) penetrated by micropores.

Replication:

- Mitosis: usually closed with an intranuclear spindle; in some species it is open at the poles
- Cell division: usually by schizogony
- Meiosis: Occurs in the zygote

General Features

Within this phylum there are three groups - coccidians, gregarines and haemosporidians. The coccidians and gregarines appear to be relatively closely related. *Perkinsus* while once considered a member of this phylum has been moved to a new phylum - *Perkinsozoa*.

Gregarines

The gregarines are generally parasites of annelids, arthropods and mollusks. They are often found in the guts of their hosts but may invade the other tissues. In the typical gregarine life cycle a trophozoite develops within a host cell into a plasmodium. This then divides into a number of merozoites by schizogony. The merozoites are released by lysing the host cell which in turn invade other cells. At some point in the life cycle gamonts are formed. These are released by lysis of the host cells and group together by syzygy. Each gamont forms multiple gametes. The gametes fuse with another to form oocysts. The oocysts leave the host to be taken up by a new host.

Coccidians

Coccidians are generally parasites of vertebrates. Like gregarines they are commonly parasites of the epithelial cells of the gut but may infect other tissues. The typical coccidial life cycle while similar to that of the gregarines differs in zygote formation. Some trophozoites enlage and become macrogamete while others divide repeatedly to form microgametes. The microgametes are motile and must reach the macrogamete to fertilize it. The fertilized macrogamete forms a zygote which in its turn forms an oocyst which is normally released from the body.

Haemosporidia

The Haemosporidians have more complex life cycles that alternate between an arthropod and a vertebrate host. The trophozoite parasitises erythrocytes or other tissues in the vertebrate host. Microgametes and macrogametes are always found in the blood. The gametes are taken up by the insect vector during a blood meal. The microgametes migrate within the gut of the insect vector and fuse with the macrogametes. The fertilized macrogamete now becomes an ookinete which penetrates the body of the vector. The ookinete then transforms into an oocyst and divides initially by meiosis and then by mitosis (haplontic life cycle) to give rise to the sporozoites. The sporozoites escape from the oocyst and migrate within the body of the vector to the salivary glands where they are injected into the new vertebrate host when the insect vector feeds again.

Blood-Borne Genera

Within the Apicomplexa there are three suborders of parasites.

- suborder Adeleorina - 8 genera
- suborder Haemosporina - all genera in this suborder
- suborder Eimeriorina - 2 genera (*Lankesterella* and *Schellackia*)

Within the *Adelorina* are species that infect invertebrates and others that infect vertebrates. The *Haemosporina* includes the malaria parasites and their relatives. The *Eimeriorina* - the largest suborder in this phylum - the life cycle involves both sexual and asexual stages. The asexual stages reproduce by schizogony. The male gametocyte produces a large number of gametes and the zygote gives rise to an oocyst which is the infective stage. The majority are monoxenous (infect one host only) but a few are heteroxenous (life cycle involves two or more hosts). Both the number of families in this later suborder is debated with the number of families being between one and twenty depending on the authority and the number of genera being between nineteen and twenty five. This somewhat unsatisfactory state of affairs awaits resolution with DNA based methods.

Disease Genomics

As noted above, many of the apicomplexan parasites are important pathogens of human and domestic animals. In contrast to bacterial pathogens, these apicomplexan parasites are eukaryote and share many metabolic pathways with their animal hosts.

This fact makes therapeutic target development extremely difficult – a drug that harms an apicomplexan parasite is also likely to harm its human host. Currently there are no effective vaccines available for most diseases caused by these parasites. Biomedical research on these parasites is challenging because it is often difficult, if not impossible, to maintain live parasite cultures in the laboratory and to genetically manipulate these organisms. In the recent years, several of the apicomplexan species have been selected for genome sequencing.

The availability of genome sequences provides a new opportunity for scientists to learn more about the evolution and biochemical capacity of these parasite. One prominent source of this genomic information is the EuPathDB family of websites, which currently provide specialised services for *Plasmodium* species (PlasmoDB), coccidians (ToxoDB), piroplasms (PiroplasmaDB), and *Cryptosporidium* species (CryptoDB). One possible target for drugs is the plastid, and in fact existing drugs such as tetracyclines which are effective against apicomplexans seem to operate against the plastid. Most apicomplexans have plastid (also known as apicoplast) and mitochondrial genomes as well as nuclear ones, although *Cryptosporidium* spp. and possibly gregarines are exceptions as they are thought to have lost their plastids after the diverging last common ancestor of apicomplexans.

Myxozoa

The Myxozoa are a group of parasitic animals of aquatic environments. Over 1300 species have been described and many have a two-host lifecycle, involving a fish and an annelid worm or bryozoan. The average size of a myxosporean spore usually ranges from 10 ìm to 20 ìm whereas that of a malacosprean spore can be up to 2 mm. Infection occurs through valved spores. These contain one or two sporoblast cells and one or more polar capsules that contain filaments which anchor the spore to its host.

The sporoblasts are then released as a motile form, called an amoebula, which penetrates the host tissues and develops into one or more multinucleate plasmodia. Certain nuclei later pair up, one engulfing another, to form new spores.

Phylogenetics

The Myxozoa were originally considered protozoan, and were included among other non-motile forms in the group Sporozoa. As their distinct nature became clear through 18S ribosomal DNA (rDNA) sequencing, they were relocated in the metazoa. Further classification was hindered by conflicting evidence: although 18S rDNA suggested an affinity with Cnidaria, other rDNA sampled, and the HOX genes of two species, were more similar to those of the Bilateria.

The discovery that *Buddenbrockia plumatellae*, a worm-like parasite up to 2 mm in length, is a myxozoan appeared to strengthen the case for a bilaterian origin, as the body plan is superficially similar. Nevertheless, closer examination reveals that *Buddenbrockia* is not longitudinally symmetrical by two ways, but four, casting doubt on this hypothesis.

Further testing has sourced the first three HOX genes found in previous research (*Myx1-3*) to the bryozoan *Cristatella mucedo*, and the fourth (*Myx4*) to Northern pike. This explained the confusion; original experiments had used contaminated tissue from host organisms, leading to false positives for a position among the Bilateria.

More careful cloning of 50 coding genes from *Buddenbrockia* established the clade as severely modified members of the phylum Cnidaria, with medusozoans as their closest relatives. Similarities between myxozoan polar capsules and cnidarian nematocysts (stinging cells) had been drawn for a long time, but were generally assumed to be the result of convergent evolution (Still these are insufficient information).

Taxonomists now recognise the outdated subgroup Actinosporea as a life-cycle phase of Myxosporea.

Species

Some species of myxozoa include:

- Class Malacosporea
  - *Buddenbrockia plumatellae*
  - *Tetracapsuloides bryosalmonae* - an important salmon parasite.
- Class Myxosporea
  - *Myxobolus cerebralis* - an important parasite of salmon and trout.

Pathology

Relationships between myxosporeans and their hosts are often highly evolved and do not usually result in severe diseases. Infection in fish hosts can be extremely long-lasting, potentially persisting for the lifetime of the host, however, an increasing number of myxosporeans have been recognised as commercially important pathogens of fish, largely as a result of the recent increase in aquaculture. The economic impact of such parasites can be severe, especially where prevalence rates are high; they may also have a severe impact on wild fish stocks.

The most significant diseases worldwide caused by myxosporeas in cultured fishes are PKD-Proliferative Kidney Disease, caused by a Malacosporea member, *Tetracapsuloides bryosalmonae*, and whirling disease, caused by a Myxosporea member *Myxobolus cerebralis*; both diseases affect salmonids. Furthermore, Enteromyxosis is caused by *Enteromyxum leei* in cultured marine sparids, while "Hamburger disease" or Proliferative Gill Disease is caused by *Henneguya ictaluri* in catfish and *Sphaerosphora renicola* infections occur in common carp.

Microsporidia

The microsporidia constitute a phylum of spore-forming unicellular parasites. They were once thought to be protists but are now known to be fungi. Loosely 1500 of the probably more than one million species are named now. Microsporidia are restricted to animal hosts, and all major groups of animals host microsporidia. Most infect insects, but they are also responsible for common diseases of crustaceans and fish. The distinguished species of microsporidia usually infect one specific host or a related group of hosts. Several species, most of which are opportunistic, also infect humans. Approximately 10 percent of the species are parasites of vertebrates, including in humans.

After infection they influence their hosts in various ways and all organs and tissues are invaded. Some species are lethal, and a few are used in biological control of insect pests. Parasitic castration, gigantism, change of host sex are effects of microsporidian parasitism.

In the most advanced cases of parasitism the microsporidium rules the host cell completely and controls its metabolism and reproduction, forming a xenoma. Replication takes place within the host's cells, which are infected by means of unicellular spores. These vary from 1-40 ìm, making them some of the smallest eukaryotes. Microsporidia that infect mammals are 1.0-4.0 ìm. They also have the smallest eukaryotic genomes. Microsporidium was once the vernacular name for a member of the class Microsporidea in the protozoan subphylum Cnidospora.

Infection

In the gut of the host the spore germinates, it builds up osmotic pressure until its rigid wall ruptures at its thinnest point at the apex. The posterior vacuole swells, forcing the polar filament to rapidly eject the infectious content into the cytoplasm of the potential host. Simultaneously the material of the filament is rearranged to form a tube which functions as a hypodermic needle and penetrates the gut epithelium. Once inside the host cell, a sporoplasm grows, dividing or forming a multinucleate plasmodium, before producing new spores. The life cycle varies considerably. Some have a simple asexual life cycle, while others have a complex life cycle involving multiple hosts and both asexual and sexual reproduction. Different types of spores may be produced at different stages, probably with different functions including autoinfection (transmission within a single host).

Ciliate

The ciliates are a group of protozoans characterised by the presence of hair-like organelles called cilia, which are identical in structure to eukaryotic flagella, but typically shorter and present in much larger numbers with a different undulating pattern than flagella. Cilia occur in all members of the group (although the peculiar Suctoria only have them for part of the life-cycle) and are variously used in swimming, crawling, attachment, feeding, and sensation. Ciliates are one of the most important groups of protists, common almost everywhere there is water — in lakes, ponds, oceans, rivers, and soils. Ciliates have many ectosymbiotic and endosymbiotic members, as well as some obligate and opportunistic parasites. Ciliates are large single cells, a few reaching 2 mm in length, and are some of the most complex protozoans in structure. The term "Ciliophora" is used in classification as a phylum. Ciliophora can be classified under Protista or Protozoa. The term "Ciliata" is also used, as a class. (However, this latter term can also refer to a type of fish.) Protista classification is rapidly evolving, and it is not rare to encounter these terms used to describe other hierarchical levels.

Cell Structure

Unlike most other eukaryotes, ciliates have two different sorts of nuclei: a small, diploid micronucleus (reproduction), and a large, polyploid macronucleus (general cell regulation). The latter is generated from the micronucleus by amplification of the genome and heavy editing. Division of the macronucleus occurs by amitosis, the segregation of the chromosomes is by a process whose mechanism is unknown. This process is by no means perfect, and after about 200 generations the cell shows signs of aging. Periodically the macronuclei must be regenerated from the micronuclei. In most, this occurs during *conjugation*. Here two cells line up, the micronuclei undergo meiosis, some of the haploid daughters are exchanged and then fuse to form new micronuclei and macronuclei. Food vacuoles are formed through phagocytosis and typically follow a particular path through the cell as their contents are digested and broken down via lysosomes so the substances the vacuole contains are then small enough to diffuse through the membrane of the food vacuole into the cell. Anything left in the food vacuole by the time it reaches the cytoproct (anus) is discharged via exocytosis. Most ciliates also have one or more prominent contractile vacuoles, which collect water and expel it from the cell to maintain osmotic pressure, or in some function to maintain ionic balance. These often have a distinctive star-shape, with each point being a collecting tube.

Reproduction

Ciliates can undergo both asexual and sexual reproduction. Asexual reproduction occurs by binary fission. The micronucleus undergoes mitosis and the macronucleus elongates and splits in half. The cell then divides in two. Both new cells each obtain a copy of the micronucleus and macronucleus. By contrast, sexual reproduction involves the exchange of genetic material (or conjugation) between two organisms of different mating type (akin to sex, but more than two mating types can exist). This often occurs when food is rare. The two cells form a bridge between their cytoplasms, the micronuclei undergo meiosis, the macronuclei disappear, and the haploid micronuclei are exchanged over the bridge. The cells separate and form new macronuclei from their micronuclei. The two cells then divide, forming four new cells.

Specialised Structures in Ciliates

In some forms there are also body polykinetids, for instance, among the spirotrichs where they generally form bristles called *cirri*. More often body cilia are arranged in *mono-* and *dikinetids*, which respectively include one and two kinetosomes (basal bodies), each of which may support a cilium. These are arranged into rows called *kineties*, which run from the anterior to posterior of the cell. The body and oral kinetids make up the *infraciliature*, an organisation unique to the ciliates and important in their classification, and include various fibrils and microtubules involved in coordinating the cilia. The infraciliature is one of the main component of the cell cortex. Another are the *alveoli*, small vesicles under the cell membrane that are packed against it to form a pellicle maintaining the cell's shape, which varies from flexible and contractile to rigid. Numerous mitochondria and extrusomes are also generally present. The presence of alveoli, the structure of the cilia, the form of mitosis and various other details indicate a close relationship between the ciliates, Apicomplexa, and dinoflagellates. These superficially dissimilar groups make up the alveolates.

Fossil Record

Until recently, the oldest ciliate fossils known were tintinnids from the Ordovician Period. In 2007, Li *et al.* published a description of fossil ciliates from the Doushantuo Formation, about 580 million years ago, in the Ediacaran Period. These included two types of tintinnids and a possible ancestral suctorian.

DNA Rearrangements (Gene Scrambling)

Ciliates contain two types of nuclei: the somatic "macronucleus" and the germline "micronucleus". Only the DNA in the micronucleus is passed on during sexual reproduction (conjugation). On the other hand, only the DNA in the macronucleus is actively expressed and results in the phenotype of the organism. Macronuclear DNA is derived from micronuclear DNA by amazingly extensive DNA rearrangement and amplification. The macronucleus begins as a copy of the micronucleus. The micronuclear chromosomes are fragmented into many smaller pieces and amplified to give many copies. The resulting macronuclear chromosomes often contain only a single gene. In *Tetrahymena*, the micronucleus has 10 chromosomes (5 per haploid genome), while the macronucleus has over 20,000 chromosomes. In addition, the micronuclear genes are interrupted by numerous "Internal Eliminated Sequences" (IESs). During development of the macronucleus, IESs are deleted and the remaining gene segments, Macronuclear Destined Sequences (MDSs), are spliced together to give the operational gene. *Tetrahymena* has about 6000 IESs and about 15% of micronuclear DNA is eliminated during this process. The process is guided by small RNAs and epigenetic chromatin marks. In spirotrich ciliates (such as *Oxytricha*), the process is even more complex due to "gene scrambling": the MDSs in the micronucleus are often in different order and orientation from that in the macronuclear gene, and so in addition to deletion, DNA inversion and translocation are required for "unscrambling". This process is guided by long RNAs derived from the parental macronucleus. More than 95% of micronuclear DNA is eliminated during spirotrich macronuclear development.

Chapter 5

Human Gastrointestinal Tract

The human gastrointestinal tract is the stomach and intestine, sometimes including all the structures from the mouth to the anus. (The "digestive system" is a broader term that includes other structures, including the accessory organs of digestion). In an adult male human, the gastrointestinal (GI) tract is 5 metres (20 ft) long in a live subject, or up to 9 metres (30 ft) without the effect of muscle tone, and consists of the upper and lower GI tracts.

The tract may also be divided into foregut, midgut, and hindgut, reflecting the embryological origin of each segment of the tract. The GI tract always releases hormones to help regulate the digestion process. These hormones, including gastrin, secretin, cholecystokinin, and grehlin, are mediated through either intracrine or autocrine mechanisms, indicating that the cells releasing these hormones are conserved structures throughout evolution.

Upper Gastrointestinal Tract

The upper gastrointestinal tract consists of the esophagus, stomach, and duodenum. The exact demarcation between "upper" and "lower" can vary. Upon gross dissection, the duodenum may appear to be a unified organ, but it is often divided into two parts based upon function, arterial supply, or embryology.

Lower Gastrointestinal Tract: The lower gastrointestinal tract includes most of the small intestine and all of the large intestine. According to some sources, it also includes the anus.

- Bowel or intestine
  - o Small Intestine: Has three parts:
    - Duodenum: Here the digestive juices from the pancreas (digestive enzymes) and hormones and the gall bladder (bile) mix. The digestive enzymes break down proteins and bile and emulsify fats into micelles. The duodenum contains Brunner's glands which produce bicarbonate. In combination with bicarbonate from pancreatic juice, this neutralizes HCl of the stomach.
    - Jejunum: This is the midsection of the intestine, connecting the duodenum to the ileum. It contains the plicae circulares, and villi to increase the surface area of that part of the GI Tract. Products of digestion (sugars, amino acids, fatty acids) are absorbed into the bloodstream.
    - Ileum: Has villi and absorbs mainly vitamin B12 and bile acids, as well as any other remaining nutrients.
  - o Large Intestine: Has three parts:
    - Caecum: The Vermiform appendix is attached to the caecum.
    - Colon: Includes the ascending colon, transverse colon, descending colon and sigmoid Flexure: The main function of the Colon is to absorb water, but it also contains bacteria that produce beneficial vitamins like vitamin K.
    - Rectum
- Anus: Passes fecal matter from the body.

The Ligament of Treitz is sometimes used to divide the upper and lower GI tracts.

Embryology

The gut is an endoderm-derived structure. At approximately the sixteenth day of human development, the embryo begins to fold ventrally (with the embryo's ventral surface becoming concave) in two directions: the sides of the embryo fold in on each other and the head and tail fold toward one another. The result is that a piece of the yolk sac, an endoderm-lined structure in contact with the ventral aspect of the embryo, begins to be pinched off to become the primitive gut. The yolk sac remains connected to the gut tube via the vitelline duct. Usually this structure regresses during development; in cases where it does not, it is known as Meckel's diverticulum. During fetal life, the primitive gut can be divided into three segments: foregut, midgut, and hindgut. Although these terms are often used in reference to segments of the primitive gut, they are also used regularly to describe components of the definitive gut as well. Each segment of the gut gives rise to specific gut and gut-related structures in later development. Components derived from the gut proper, including the stomach and colon, develop as swellings or dilatations of the primitive gut. In contrast, gut-related derivatives — that is, those structures that derive from the primitive gut but are not part of the gut proper, in general develop as out-pouchings of the primitive gut. The blood vessels supplying these structures remain constant throughout development.

Transit Time

The time taken for food or other ingested objects to transit through the gastrointestinal tract varies depending on many factors, but roughly, it takes 2.5 to 3 hours after a meal for 50% of stomach contents to empty into the intestines and total emptying of the stomach takes 4 to 5 hours. Subsequently, 50% emptying of the small intestine takes 2.5 to 3 hours. Finally, transit through the colon takes 30 to 40 hours.

Pathology

There are a number of diseases and conditions affecting the gastrointestinal system, including:

- Appendicitis
- Cancer
- Celiac Disease
- Cholera
- Colorectal cancer

- Diarrhoea
- Diverticulitis
- Enteric duplication cyst
- Gastroenteritis, also known as “stomach flu”; an inflammation of the stomach and intestines
- Giardiasis
- Inflammatory bowel disease (including Crohn’s disease and ulcerative colitis)
- Irritable bowel syndrome
- Pancreatitis
- Peptic ulcer disease
- Yellow Fever

Immune Function

The gastrointestinal tract is also a prominent part of the immune system. The surface area of the digestive tract is estimated to be the surface area of a football field. With such a large exposure, the immune system must work hard to prevent pathogens from entering into blood and lymph.

The low pH (ranging from 1 to 4) of the stomach is fatal for many microorganisms that enter it. Similarly, mucus (containing IgA antibodies) neutralizes many of these microorganisms.

Other factors in the GI tract help with immune function as well, including enzymes in saliva and bile. Enzymes such as Cyp3A4, along with the antiporter activities, also are instrumental in the intestine’s role of detoxification of antigens and xenobiotics, such as drugs, involved in first pass metabolism.

Health-enhancing intestinal bacteria serve to prevent the overgrowth of potentially harmful bacteria in the gut. These two types of bacteria compete for space and “food,” as there are limited resources within the intestinal tract.

A ratio of 80-85% beneficial to 15-20% potentially harmful bacteria generally is considered normal within the intestines. Microorganisms also are kept at bay by an extensive immune system comprising the gut-associated lymphoid tissue (GALT).

Histology

The gastrointestinal tract has a form of general histology with some differences that reflect the specialisation in functional anatomy. The GI tract can be divided into four concentric layers:

- Mucosa
- Submucosa
- *Muscularis externa* (the external muscular layer)
- Adventitia or serosa.

Mucosa

The mucosa is the innermost layer of the gastrointestinal tract. that is surrounding the lumen, or open space within the tube. This layer comes in direct contact with digested food (chyme),

The Mucosa is Made up of Three Layers:

- Epithelium - innermost layer. Responsible for most digestive, absorptive and secretory processes.
- Lamina propria - a layer of connective tissue. Unusually cellular compared to most connective tissue
- Muscularis mucosae - a thin layer of smooth muscle. Function is still under debate

The mucosae are highly specialised in each organ of the gastrointestinal tract to deal with the different conditions. The most variation is seen in the epithelium. In the oesophagus, the epithelium is stratified, squamous and non-keratinising, for protective purposes. In the stomach it is simple columnar, and is organised into gastric pits and glands to deal with secretion. The gastro-oesophageal junction is extremely abrupt.

The small intestine epithelium (particularly the ileum) is specialised for absorption; it is organised into plicae circulares and villi, and the enterocytes have microvilli. This creates a brush border which greatly increases the surface area for absorption. The epithelium is simple columnar with microvilli. In the ileum there are occasionally Peyer's patches in the lamina propria. The colon has simple columnar epithelium with no villi. There are goblet cells. The appendix has a mucosa resembling the colon but is heavily infiltrated with lymphocytes.

The ano-rectal junction (at the pectinate line) is again very abrupt; there is a transition from simple columnar to stratified squamous non-keratinising epithelium (as in the oesophagus) for protective purposes.

Submucosa

The submucosa consists of a dense irregular layer of connective tissue with large blood vessels, lymphatics, and nerves branching into the mucosa and muscularis externa. It contains Meissner's plexus, an enteric nervous plexus, situated on the inner surface of the *muscularis externa.*

Muscularis Externa

The muscularis externa consists of an inner circular layer and a longitudinal outer muscular layer. The circular muscle layer prevents food from traveling backward and the longitudinal layer shortens the tract. The layers are not truly longitudinal or circular, rather the layers of muscle are helical with different pitches. The inner circular is helical with a steep pitch and the outer longitudinal is helical with a much shallower pitch. The coordinated contractions of these layers is called peristalsis and propels the food through the tract. Food in the GI tract is called a bolus (ball of food) from the mouth down to the stomach. After the stomach, the food is partially digested and semi-liquid, and is referred to as chyme. In the large intestine the remaining semi-solid substance is referred to as faeces.

Between the two muscle layers are the myenteric or Auerbach's plexus. This controls peristalsis. Activity is initiated by the pacemaker cells (interstitial cells of Cajal). The gut has intrinsic peristaltic activity (basal electrical rhythm) due to its self-contained enteric nervous system. The rate can of course be modulated by the rest of the autonomic nervous system.

The thickness of muscularis externa varies in each part of the tract. In the colon, for example, the muscularis externa is much thicker because the faeces are large and heavy, and require more force to push along. The outer longitudinal layer of the colon thins out into 3 discontinuous longitudinal bands, known as tiniae coli (bands of the colon). This is one of the 3 features helping to distinguish between the large and small intestine.

Occasionally in the large intestine (2-3 times a day) there will be mass contraction of certain segments, moving a lot of faeces along. This is generally when one gets the urge to defecate. The pylorus of the stomach has a thickened portion of the inner circular layer: the pyloric sphincter. Alone among the GI tract, the stomach has a third layer of muscularis externa. This is the inner oblique layer, and helps churn the chyme in the stomach.

Adventitia/serosa

The outermost layer of the GI tract consists of several layers of connective tissue. Intraperitoneal parts of the GI tract are covered with serosa. These include most of the stomach, first part of the duodenum, all of the small intestine, caecum and appendix, transverse colon, sigmoid colon and rectum. In these sections of the gut there is clear boundary between the gut and the surrounding tissue. These parts of the tract have a mesentery. Retroperitoneal parts are covered with adventitia. They blend in to the surrounding tissue and are fixed in position. For example, the retroperitoneal section of the duodenum usually passes through the transpyloric plane. These include the oesophagus, pylorus of the stomach, distal duodenum, ascending colon, descending colon and anal canal. In addition, the oral cavity has adventitia.

Human Mouth

In human anatomy, the mouth is the first portion of the alimentary canal that receives food and saliva. The oral mucosa is the mucous membrane epithelium lining the inside of the mouth. In addition to its primary role as the beginning of the digestive system, in humans the mouth also plays a significant role in communication. While primary aspects of the voice are produced in the throat, the tongue, lips, and jaw are also needed to produce the range of sounds included in human language. The mouth, normally moist, is lined with a mucous membrane, and contains the teeth. The lips mark the transition from mucous membrane to skin, which covers most of the body.

Description

Mouth Cavity: The first space of the mouth is the mouth cavity, bounded laterally and in front by the alveolar process (containing the teeth), posteriorily by the isthmus of the fauces, superiorly or the roof is formed by hard palate and soft palate and inferiorly or the floor of the mouth is formed by the mylohyoid muscles and is occupied mainly by the tongue.

The oral cavity is also known as the mouth which swallows food that then goes down the esophagus and into the stomach.

Orifice: While shut, the orifice of the mouth forms a line between the upper and lower lip.

In facial expression, this *mouth line* is iconically shaped like an up-open parabola in a smile, and like a down-open parabola in a frown. A *down-turned mouth* means a mouth line forming a down-turned parabola, and when permanent can be normal. Also, a *down-turned mouth* can be part of the presentation of Prader-Willi syndrome.

Function: The mouth plays an important role in eating, drinking and breathing. Infants are born with a sucking reflex, by which they instinctively know to suck for nourishment using their lips and jaw.

Development: The philtrum is the vertical groove in the upper lip, formed where the nasomedial and maxillary processes meet during embryo development. When these processes fail to fuse fully, a hare lip and/or cleft palate can result.

This can result in the encouraging process of the release of metabolic wastes. The nasolabial folds are the deep creases of tissue that extend from the nose to the sides of the mouth. One of the first signs of age on the human face is the increase in prominence of the nasolabial folds.

Cultural Aspects

Lips can be adorned with lipstick or lip gloss, although in most cultures, this is typically only practiced by females. Both men and women, however, apply lip balm in order to soothe chapped or dry lips. Piercings in or around the mouth have been made popular by younger generations, including those on the lip or tongue. The uvula piercing, while increasing in popularity, remains relatively rare.

Oral sex is a form of sexual intercourse practised with the mouth. Kisses are performed using the mouth.

Human Pharynx

The human pharynx (plural: *pharynges*) is the part of the throat situated immediately inferior to (below) the mouth and nasal cavity, and superior to the esophagus and larynx.

The human pharynx is conventionally divided into three sections: the nasopharynx (epipharynx), the oropharynx (mesopharynx), and the laryngopharynx (hypopharynx). The pharynx is part of the digestive system and also the respiratory system; it is also important in vocalization.

Nasopharynx

The most cephalad portion of the pharynx. It extends from the base of the skull to the upper surface of the soft palate. It includes the space between the internal nares and the soft palate and lies superior to the oral cavity. The pharyngeal tonsils, more commonly referred to as the *adenoids*, are lymphoid tissue structures located in the posterior wall of the nasopharynx.

Polyps or mucus can obstruct the nasopharynx, as can congestion due to an upper respiratory infection. The Eustachian tubes, which connect the middle ear to the pharynx, open into the nasopharynx. The opening and closing of the Eustachian tubes serves to equalize the barometric pressure in the middle ear with that of the ambient atmosphere.

The anterior aspect of the nasopharynx communicates through the choanae with the nasal cavities. On its lateral walls are the pharyngeal ostia of the auditory tube, somewhat triangular in shape, and bounded behind by a firm prominence, the torus tubarius or cushion, caused by the medial end of the cartilage of the tube that elevates the mucous membrane. Two folds arise from the cartilaginous opening:

- the salpingopharyngeal fold, a vertical fold of mucous membrane extending from the inferior part of the torus and containing the salpingopharyngeus muscle
- the salpingopalatine fold, a smaller fold extending from the superior part of the torus to the palate and containing the levator veli palatini muscle. The tensor veli palatini is lateral to the levator and does not contribute the fold, since the origin is deep to the cartilaginous opening.

Behind the ostium of the auditory tube is a deep recess, the pharyngeal recess (also referred to as the *fossa of Rosenmüller*). On the posterior wall is a prominence, best marked in childhood, produced by a mass of lymphoid tissue, which is known as the pharyngeal tonsil. Superior to the pharyngeal tonsil, in the midline, an irregular flask-shaped depression of the mucous membrane sometimes extends up as far as the basilar process of the occipital bone; it is known as the *pharyngeal bursa*.

Oropharynx

The oropharynx or mesopharynx lies behind the oral cavity, extending from the uvula to the level of the hyoid bone. It opens anteriorly, through the isthmus faucium, into the mouth, while in its lateral wall, between the Palatoglossal arch and the Palatopharyngeal arch, is the palatine tonsil. The anterior wall consists of the base of the tongue and the epiglottic vallecula; the lateral wall is made up of the tonsil, tonsillar fossa, and tonsillar (faucial) pillars; the superior wall consists of the inferior surface of the soft palate and the uvula. Because both food and air pass through the pharynx, a flap of connective tissue called the epiglottis closes over the glottis when food is swallowed to prevent aspiration. The oropharynx is lined by non keratinised squamous stratified epithelium.

The *HACEK* organisms (*Haemophilus, Actinobacillus actinomycetemcomitans, Cardiobacterium hominis, Eikenella corrodens, Kingella*) are part of the normal oropharyngeal flora, which grow slowly, prefer a carbon dioxide-enriched atmosphere, and share an enhanced capacity to produce endocardial infections, especially in young children. *Fusobacterium* is a pathogen.

Laryngopharynx

The hypopharynx or laryngopharynx or (Latin: *pars laryngea pharyngis*) is the caudal part of the pharynx; it is the part of the throat that connects to the esophagus. It lies inferior to the epiglottis and extends to the location where this common pathway diverges into the respiratory (larynx) and digestive (esophagus) pathways. At that point, the laryngopharynx is continuous with the esophagus posteriorly. The esophagus conducts food and fluids to the stomach; air enters the larynx anteriorly. During swallowing, food has the "right of way", and air passage temporarily stops.

Corresponding roughly to the area located between the 4th and 6th cervical vertebrae, the superior boundary of the laryngopharynx is at the level of the hyoid bone. The laryngopharynx includes three major sites: the pyriform sinus, postcricoid area, and the posterior pharyngeal wall. Like the oropharynx above it, the laryngopharynx serves as a passageway for food and air and is lined with a stratified squamous epithelium. It is innervated by the pharyngeal plexus.

Stomach

The stomach is a muscular, hollow, dilated part of the digestion system which functions as an important organ of the digestive tract in some animals, including vertebrates, echinoderms, insects (mid-gut), and molluscs. It is involved in the second phase of digestion, following mastication (chewing).

The stomach is located between the esophagus and the small intestine. It secretes protein-digesting enzymes called protease and strong acids to aid in food digestion, (sent to it via oesophageal peristalsis) through smooth muscular contortions (called segmentation) before sending partially digested food (chyme) to the small intestines.

The word *stomach* is derived from the Latin *stomachus* which is derived from the Greek word *stomachos*, ultimately from *stoma* (óôüìá), "mouth". The words *gastro-* and *gastric* (meaning related to the stomach) are both derived from the Greek word *gaster* (ãáóôÞñ).

Role in Digestion

Bolus (masticated food) enters the stomach through the oesophagus via the oesophageal sphincter. The stomach releases proteases (protein-digesting enzymes such as pepsin) and hydrochloric acid, which kills or inhibits bacteria and provides the acidic pH of two for the proteases to work. Food is churned by the stomach through muscular contractions of the wall called peristalsis – reducing the volume of the fundus, before looping around the fundus and the body of stomach as the boluses are converted into chyme (partially digested food). Chyme slowly passes through the pyloric sphincter and into the duodenum of the small intestine, where the extraction of nutrients begins. Depending on the quantity and contents of the meal, the stomach will digest the food into chyme anywhere between forty minutes and a few hours. The average human stomach can comfortably hold about a litre of food.

Gastric juice in the stomach also contains pepsinogen and prorennin. Hydrochloric acid activates these inactive forms of enzymes into active forms which are pepsin and renin (proteases). Rennin digests the milk protein Caesinogen (soluble) into caesin (insoluble) thus curdling the milk. Pepsin breaks down proteins into polypeptides.

Anatomy of the Stomach

The stomach lies between the esophagus and the duodenum (the first part of the small intestine). It is on the left upper part of the abdominal cavity. The top of the stomach lies against the diaphragm. Lying behind the stomach is the pancreas. The greater omentum hangs down from the *greater curvature.*

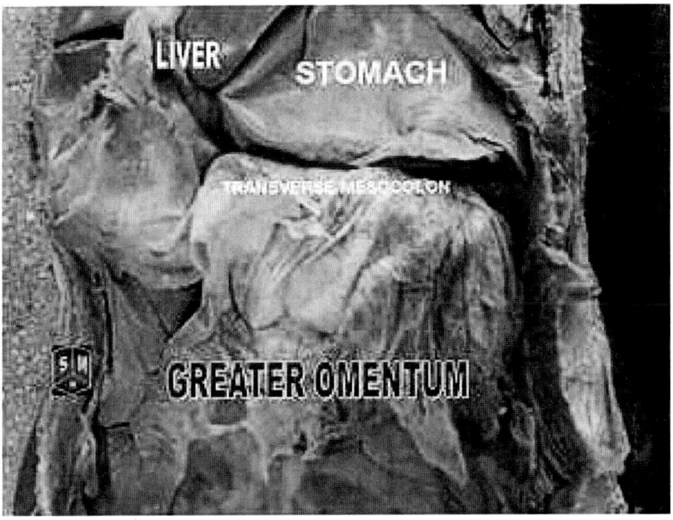

Figure: *Greater omentum and stomach*

Two sphincters keep the contents of the stomach contained. They are the esophageal sphincter (found in the cardiac region, not an anatomical sphincter) dividing the tract above, and the Pyloric sphincter dividing the stomach from the small intestine.

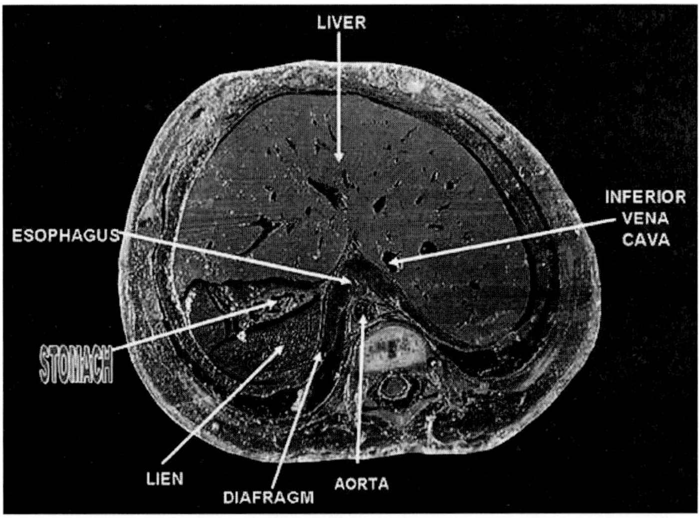

Figure: *Stomach*

The stomach is surrounded by parasympathetic (stimulant) and orthosympathetic (inhibitor) plexuses (networks of blood vessels and nerves in the anterior gastric, posterior, superior and inferior, celiac and myenteric), which regulate both the secretions activity and the motor (motion) activity of its muscles.

In adult humans, the stomach has a relaxed, near empty volume of about 45 to 75 ml. Because it is a distensible organ, it normally expands to hold about one litre of food, but can hold as much as two to three litres. The stomach of a newborn human baby will only be able to retain about 30 ml.

Control of Secretion and Motility

The movement and the flow of chemicals into the stomach are controlled by both the autonomic nervous system and by the various digestive system hormones:

Gastrin	The hormone *gastrin* causes an increase in the secretion of HCl from the parietal cells, and pepsinogen from chief cells in the stomach. It also causes increased motility in the stomach. Gastrin is released by G-cells in the stomach in response to distenstion of the antrum, and digestive products (especially large quantities of incompletely digested proteins). It is inhibited

	by a pH normally less than 4 (high acid), as well as the hormone somatostatin.
Cholecystokinin	*Cholecystokinin* (CCK) has most effect on the gall bladder, causing gall bladder contractions, but it also decreases gastric emptying and increases release of pancreatic juice which is alkaline and neutralizes the chyme.
Secretin	In a different and rare manner, *secretin*, produced in the small intestine, has most effects on the pancreas, but will also diminish acid secretion in the stomach.
Gastric inhibitory peptide	*Gastric inhibitory peptide* (GIP) decreases both gastric acid release and motility.
Enteroglucagon	*enteroglucagon* decreases both gastric acid and motility.

Other than gastrin, these hormones all act to turn off the stomach action. This is in response to food products in the liver and gall bladder, which have not yet been absorbed. The stomach needs to push food into the small intestine only when the intestine is not busy. While the intestine is full and still digesting food, the stomach acts as storage for food.

EGF in gastric defence

Epidermal growth factor (EGF) results in cellular proliferation, differentiation, and survival. EGF is a low-molecular-weight polypeptide first purified from the mouse submandibular gland, but since then found in many human tissues including submandibular gland, parotid gland. Salivary EGF, which seems also regulated by dietary inorganic iodine, plays also an important physiological role in the maintenance of oro-oesophageal and gastric tissue integrity. The biological effects of salivary EGF include healing of oral and gastroesophageal ulcers, inhibition of gastric acid secretion, stimulation of DNA synthesis as well as mucosal protection from intraluminal injurious factors such as gastric acid, bile acids, pepsin, and trypsin and to physical, chemical and bacterial agents.

Stomach as Nutrition Sensor

The stomach can "taste" sodium glutamate using glutamate receptors and this information is passed to the lateral hypothalamus and limbic system in the brain as a palatability signal through the vagus nerve. The stomach can also sense independently to tongue and oral taste receptors glucose, carbohydrates proteins, and fats. This allows the brain to link nutritional value of foods to their tastes.

Absorption

Although the absorption is mainly a function of the small intestine, some absorption of certain small molecules nevertheless does occur in the stomach through its lining. This includes:

- Water, if the body is dehydrated
- Medication, like aspirin
- Amino acids
- 10-20% of ingested ethanol (e.g. from alcoholic beverages)
- Caffeine.

Diseases of the Stomach

A large number of studies have indicated that most cases of peptic ulcers, gastritis, and stomach cancer are caused by *Helicobacter pylori* infection. The stomach has to regenerate a new layer of mucus every two weeks, or else damage to the epithelium may result.

In Other Animals

Although the precise shape and size of the stomach varies widely among different vertebrates, the relative positions of the oesophageal and duodenal openings remain relatively constant. As a result, the organ always curves somewhat to the left before curving back to meet the pyloric sphincter. However, lampreys, hagfishes, chimaeras, lungfishes, and some teleost fish have no stomach at all, with the oesophagus opening directly into the intestine. These animals all consume diets that either require little storage of food, or no pre-digestion with gastric juices, or both. The gastric lining is usually divided into two regions, an anterior portion lined by fundic glands, and a posterior with pyloric glands. Cardiac glands are unique to mammals, and even then are absent in a number of species. The distributions of these glands vary between species, and do not always correspond with the same regions as in man.

Furthermore, in many non-human mammals, a portion of the stomach anterior to the cardiac glands is lined with epithelium essentially identical to that of the oesophagus. Ruminants, in particular, have a complex stomach, the first three chambers of which are all lined with oesophageal mucosa. In birds and crocodilians, the stomach is divided into two regions. Anteriorly is a narrow tubular region, the proventriculus, lined by fundic glands, and connecting the true stomach to the crop. Beyond lies the powerful muscular gizzard, lined by pyloric glands, and, in some species, containing stones that the animal swallows to help grind up food.

Small Intestine

The small intestine (or small bowel) is the part of the gastrointestinal tract following the stomach and followed by the large intestine, and is where much of the digestion and absorption of food takes place. In invertebrates such as worms, the terms "gastrointestinal tract" and "large intestine" are often used to describe the entire intestine. This article is primarily about the human gut, though the information about its processes is directly applicable to most placental mammals. The primary function of the small intestine is the absorption of nutrients and minerals found in food. (A major exception to this is cows; for information about digestion in cows and other similar mammals.)

Size and Divisions

The average length of the small intestine in an adult human male is 6.9 m (22 feet 6 inches), and in the adult female 7.1 m (23 feet 4 inches). It can vary greatly, from as short as 4.6 m (15 feet) to as long as 9.8 m (32 feet). It is approximately 2.5–3 cm in diametre. The small intestine is divided into three structural parts:

Duodenum

The duodenum is the first section of the small intestine in most higher vertebrates, including mammals, reptiles, and birds. In fish, the divisions of the small intestine are not as clear, and the terms anterior intestine or proximal intestine may be used instead of duodenum. In mammals the duodenum may be the principal site for iron absorption.

The duodenum precedes the jejunum and ileum and is the shortest part of the small intestine, where most chemical digestion takes place. The name *duodenum* is from the Latin *duodenum digitorum*, or "twelve fingers' breadth". In humans, the duodenum is a hollow jointed tube about 25-38cm (10-15 inches) long connecting the stomach to the jejunum. It begins with the duodenal bulb and ends at the ligament of Treitz.

Function

The duodenum is largely responsible for the breakdown of food in the small intestine, using enzymes. Brunner's glands, which secrete mucus, are found in the duodenum. The duodenum wall is composed of a very thin layer of cells that form the muscularis mucosae. The duodenum is almost entirely retroperitoneal. The duodenum also regulates the rate of emptying of the stomach via hormonal pathways. Secretin and cholecystokinin are released from cells in the duodenal epithelium in response to acidic and fatty stimuli present there when the pylorus opens and releases gastric chyme into the duodenum for further digestion. These cause the liver and gall bladder to release bile, and the pancreas to release bicarbonate and digestive enzymes such as trypsin, lipase and amylase into the duodenum as they are needed.

Sections

The duodenum is divided into four sections for the purposes of description. The first three sections curve in a "C"-loop concavity in which the head of the pancreas lies. Only the first 2 cm of the superior part is mobile (covered by peritoneum) – the distal 3 cm of the first part along with the rest of the duodenum is retroperitoneal (immobile).

First Part

The first (superior) part begins as a continuation of the duodenal end of the pylorus. From here it passes laterally (right), superiorly and posteriorly, for approximately 5 cm, before making a sharp curve inferiorly into the superior duodenal flexure (the end of the superior part). It is the only intraperitoneal portion of the duodenum. Relations:

- Anterior
    - o Gallbladder

    - o Quadrate lobe of liver
- Posterior
    - o Bile duct
    - o Gastroduodenal artery
    - o Portal vein
    - o Inferior vena cava
    - o Head of pancreas
- Superior
    - o Neck of gallbladder
    - o Hepatoduodenal ligament (lesser omentum)
- Inferior
    - o Neck of pancreas
    - o Greater omentum
    - o Head of pancreas.

Second Part

The second (descending) part of the duodenum begins at the superior duodenal flexure. It passes inferiorly to the lower border of vertebral body L3, before making a sharp turn medially into the inferior duodenal flexure (the end of the descending part).

The pancreatic duct and common bile duct enter the descending duodenum, commonly known together as the hepatopancreatic duct (or pancreatic duct in the United States), through the major duodenal papilla (known as Ampulla of Vater).

This part of the duodenum also contains the minor duodenal papilla, the entrance for the accessory pancreatic duct (of Santorini). The junction between the embryological foregut and midgut lies just below the major duodenal papilla.

Third Part

The third (inferior/horizontal) part of the duodenum begins at the inferior duodenal flexure and passes transversely to the left, crossing the right ureter, right testicular/ovarian vessels, inferior vena cava, abdominal aorta, superior mesenteric artery and the vertebral column.

Fourth Part

The fourth (ascending) part passes superiorly, either anterior to, or to the left of, the aorta, until it reaches the inferior border of the body of the pancreas. Then, it curves anteriorly and terminates at the duodenojejunal flexure where it joins the jejunum. The duodenojejunal flexure is surrounded by a peritoneal fold containing muscle fibres: the ligament of Treitz.

Blood Supply

The duodenum receives arterial blood from two different sources. The transition between these sources is important as it demarcates the foregut from the midgut. Proximal to the 2nd part of the duodenum (approximately at the major duodenal papilla – where the bile duct enters) the arterial supply is from the gastroduodenal artery and its branch the superior pancreaticoduodenal artery. Distal to this point (the midgut) the arterial supply is from the superior mesenteric artery (SMA), and its branch the inferior pancreaticoduodenal artery supplies the 3rd and 4th sections. The superior and inferior pancreaticoduodenal arteries (from the gastroduodenal artery and SMA respectively) form an anastomotic loop between the celiac trunk and the SMA; so there is potential for collateral circulation here. The venous drainage of the duodenum follows the arteries. Ultimately these veins drain into the portal system, either directly or indirectly through the splenic or superior mesenteric vein.

Lymphatic Drainage

The lymphatic vessels follow the arteries in a retrograde fashion. The anterior lymphatic vessels drain into the pancreatoduodenal lymph nodes located along the superior and inferior pancreatoduodenal arteries and then into the pyloric lymph nodes (along the gastroduodenal artery). The posterior lymphatic vessels pass posterior to the head of the pancreas and drain into the superior mesenteric lymph nodes. Efferent lymphatic vessels from the duodenal lymph nodes ultimately pass into the celiac lymph nodes.

Jejunum

The jejunum is the middle section of the small intestine in most higher vertebrates, including mammals, reptiles, and birds. In fish, the divisions of the small intestine are not as clear and the terms middle intestine or mid-gut may be used instead of jejunum. The jejunum lies between the duodenum and the ileum. The change from the duodenum to the jejunum is usually defined as the Duodenojejunal flexure and is attached, and thus "hung up", to the ventricle by the ligament of Treitz. In adult humans, the small intestine is usually between 5.5 and 6m long, 2.5m of which is the jejunum. The pH in the jejunum is usually between 7 and 9 (neutral or slightly alkaline). If the jejunum is impacted by blunt force the emesis reflex will be initiated. The jejunum and the ileum are suspended by mesentery which gives the bowel great mobility within the abdomen. It also contains circular and longitudinal smooth muscle which helps to move food along by a process known as peristalsis.

Function

The jejunum is the second portion of the small intestine, and it has a lining which is specialised in the absorption of monosaccharides (fully digested carbohydrates) and amino acids (fully digested proteins). The proteins have been broken down in the stomach by acid and an enzyme called pepsin into amino acids. The carbohydrates are broken down in the duodenum by enzymes from the pancreas and liver into sugars.

Fats are broken down in the duodenum by "lipase" from the pancreas into fatty acids. Amino acid, sugar, fatty acid particles, vitamins, minerals, electrolytes and water are small enough to soak into the villi of the jejunum and drop into the blood stream. The blood takes all these nutrients to all the other parts of the body to provide fuel to do their jobs.

Internal Structure

The inner surface of the jejunum, its mucous membrane, is covered in projections called villi, which increase the surface area of tissue available to absorb nutrients from the gut contents. The epithelial cells which line these villi possess even larger numbers of microvilli. The transport of nutrients across epithelial cells through the jejunum and ileum includes the passive transport of sugar fructose and the active transport of amino acids, small peptides, vitamins, and most glucose.

The villi in the jejunum are much longer than in the duodenum or ileum. The jejunum contains very few Brunner's glands (found in the duodenum) or Peyer's patches (found in the ileum).

However, there are a few jejunal lymph nodes suspended in its mesentery. The jejunum has many large circular folds in its submucosa called plicae circulares which increase the surface area for nutrient absorption.

Differences Between Jejunum and Ileum

There is no line of demarcation between the jejunum and the ileum. There are, however, subtle differences between the two.

- The ileum has more fat inside the mesentery than the jejunum.
- The ileum has a paler colour, and tends to be of a smaller caliber as well.
- While the length of the intestinal tract contains lymphoid tissue, only the ileum has abundant Peyer's patches, unencapsulated lymphoid nodules that contain large numbers of lymphocytes and other cells of the immune system.

Etymology

Jejunum is derived from the Latin word *jçjûnus*, meaning "fasting". It was so called because this part of the small intestine was frequently found to be void of food following death, thanks to intensive peristaltic activity compared to the duodenum and ileum. The Early Modern English adjective *jejune* is derived from this word.

Function

The function of the ileum is mainly to absorb vitamin B_{12} and bile salts and whatever products of digestion that were not absorbed by the jejunum.

The wall itself is made up of folds, each of which has many tiny finger-like projections known as villi on its surface. In turn, the epithelial cells that line these villi possess even larger numbers of microvilli. Therefore the ileum has an extremely large surface area both for the adsorption (attachment) of enzyme molecules and for the absorption of products of digestion.

The DNES (diffuse neuroendocrine system) cells of the ileum secrete various hormones (gastrin, secretin, cholecystokinin) into the blood. Cells in the lining of the ileum secrete the protease and carbohydrase enzymes responsible for the final stages of protein and carbohydrate digestion into the lumen of the intestine.

These enzymes are present in the cytoplasm of the epithelial cells. The villi contain large numbers of capillaries that take the amino acids and glucose produced by digestion to the hepatic portal vein and the liver. Lacteals are small lymph vessels, and are present in villi. They absorb fatty acid and glycerol, the products of fat digestion. Layers of circular and longitudinal smooth muscle enable the digested food to be pushed along the ileum by waves of muscle contractions called peristalsis. The undigested food (waste and water) are sent to the colon.

Differences Between Jejunum and Ileum

There is no line of demarcation between the jejunum and the ileum. There are, however, subtle differences between the two.

- The ileum has more fat inside the mesentery than the jejunum
- The ileum has a mesenteric and an anti-mesenteric vascular supply, while the jejunum has only a mesenteric vasculature
- While the length of the intestinal tract contains lymphoid tissue, only the ileum has abundant Peyer's patches, unencapsulated lymphoid nodules that contain large numbers of lymphocytes and other cells of the immune system.

Embryology

In the fetus the ileum is connected to the navel by the vitelline duct. In roughly 2% of humans, this duct fails to close during the first seven weeks after birth, causing a condition called Meckel's diverticulum.

Veterinary Anatomy

In veterinary anatomy, the ileum is distinguished from the jejunum by being that portion of the jejunoileum that is connected to the caecum by the ileocecal fold. The ileum is the short terminal part of the small intestine and forms the connection to the large intestine. It is suspended by the caudal part of the mesentery (mesoileum) and is attached, in addition, to the cecum by the ileocecal fold. The ileum terminates at the cecocolic junction of the large intestine forming the ileal orifice. In the dog the ileal orifice is located at the level of the first or second lumbar vertebra, in the ox in the level of the fourth lumbar vertebrae, in the sheep and goat at the level of the caudal point of the costal arch. By active muscular contraction of the ileum, and closure of the ileal opening as a result of engorgement, the ileum prevents the backflow of ingesta and the equalization of pressure between jejunum and the base of the cecum. Disturbance of this sensitive balance is not uncommon and is one of the causes of colic in horses.

Large Intestine

The large intestine (or large bowel) is the last part of the digestive system in vertebrate animals. Its function is to absorb water from the remaining indigestible food matter, and then to pass useless waste material from the body. This article is primarily about the human gut, though the information about its processes are directly applicable to most mammals.

The large intestine consists of the cecum, colon, rectum and anal canal. It starts in the right iliac region of the pelvis, just at or below the right waist, where it is joined to the bottom end of the small intestine. From here it continues up the abdomen, then across the width of the abdominal cavity, and then it turns down, continuing to its endpoint at the anus.

The large intestine is about 4.9 feet (1.5 m) long, which is about one-fifth of the whole length of the intestinal canal.

In Terminologia Anatomica the large intestine includes the cecum, colon, rectum, and anal canal. However, some sources exclude the anal canal.

Function and Relation to Other Organs

The large intestine takes about 16 hours to finish the digestion of the food. It removes water and any remaining absorbable nutrients from the food before sending the indigestible matter to the Rectum. The colon absorbs vitamins which are created by the colonic bacteria - such as vitamin K (especially important as the daily ingestion of vitamin K is not normally enough to maintain adequate blood coagulation), vitamin B12, thiamine and riboflavin. It also compacts feces, and stores fecal matter in the rectum until it can be discharged via the anus in defecation.

The large intestine differs in physical form from the small intestine in being much wider and in showing the longitudinal layer of the muscularis have been reduced to 3 strap-like structures known as the taeniae coli. The wall of the large intestine is lined with simple columnar epithelium. Instead of having the evaginations of the small intestine (villi), the large intestine has invaginations (the intestinal glands). While both the small intestine and the large intestine have goblet cells, they are abundant in the large intestine.

The appendix is attached to its inferior surface of the cecum. It contains the least of lymphoid tissue. It is a part of mucosa-associated lymphoid tissue, which gives the appendix an important role in immunity. Appendicitis is the result of a blockage that traps infectious material in the lumen.

The appendix can be removed with no apparent damage or consequence to the patient. The large intestine extends from the ileocecal junction to the anus and is about 4.9 ft long. On the surface, bands of longitudinal muscle fibres called taeniae coli, each about 1/5 in wide, can be identified.

There are three bands, and they start at the base of the appendix and extend from the cecum to the rectum. Along the sides of the taeniae, tags of peritoneum filled with fat, called epiploic appendages (or appendices epiploicae) are found. The sacculations, called haustra, are characteristic features of the large intestine, and distinguish it from the small intestine.

Parts and Location

Parts of the large intestine are:

Cecum – the first part of the large intestine

- *Taeniae coli* – three bands of smooth muscle
- *Haustra* – bulges caused by contraction of taeniae coli
- *Epiploic appendages* – small fat accumulations on the viscera.

Locations along the colon are:

- The ascending colon
- The right colic flexure (hepatic)
- The transverse colon
- The transverse mesocolon
- The left colic flexure (splenic)
- The descending colon
- *The sigmoid colon* – the v-shaped region of the large intestine.

Bacterial Flora

The large intestine houses over 700 species of bacteria that perform a variety of functions. The large intestine absorbs some of the products formed by the bacteria inhabiting this region. Undigested polysaccharides (fibre) are metabolized to short-chain fatty acids by bacteria in the large intestine and absorbed by passive diffusion.

The bicarbonate that the large intestine secretes helps to neutralize the increased acidity resulting from the formation of these fatty acids.

These bacteria also produce large amounts of vitamins, especially vitamin K and biotin (a B vitamin), for absorption into the blood. Although this source of vitamins, in general, provides only a small part of the daily requirement, it makes a significant contribution when dietary vitamin intake is low.

An individual that depends on absorption of vitamins formed by bacteria in the large intestine may become vitamin-deficient if treated with antibiotics that inhibit other species of bacteria as well as the disease-causing bacteria.

Other bacterial products include gas (flatus), which is a mixture of nitrogen and carbon dioxide, with small amounts of the gases hydrogen, methane, and hydrogen sulphide. Bacterial fermentation of undigested polysaccharides produces these. The normal flora is also essential in the development of certain tissues, including the cecum and lymphatics. They are also involved in the production of cross-reactive antibodies. These are antibodies produced by the immune system against the normal flora, that are also effective against related pathogens, thereby preventing infection or invasion. The most prevalent bacteria are the bacteroides, which have been implicated in the initiation of colitis and colon cancer.

Bifidobacteria are also abundant, and are often described as 'friendly bacteria'. A mucus layer protects the large intestine from attacks from colonic commensal bacteria.

In Other Animals

The large intestine is truly distinct only in tetrapods, in which it is almost always separated from the small intestine by an ileocaecal valve. In most vertebrates, however, it is a relatively short structure running directly to the anus, although noticeably wider than the small intestine. Although the caecum is present in most amniotes, only in mammals does the remainder of the large intestine develop into a true colon.

In some small mammals, the colon is straight, as it is in other tetrapods, but, in the majority of mammalian species, it is divided into ascending and descending portions; a distinct transverse colon is typically present only in primates. However, the taeniae coli and accompanying haustra are not found in either carnivorans or ruminants. The rectum of mammals (other than monotremes) is derived from the cloaca of other vertebrates, and is, therefore, not truly homologous with the "rectum" found in these species.

In fish, there is no true large intestine, but simply a short rectum connecting the end of the digestive part of the gut to the cloaca. In sharks, this includes a *rectal gland* that secretes salt to help the animal maintain osmotic balance with the seawater. The gland somewhat resembles a caecum in structure, but is not a homologous structure.

Breakdown into Nutrients

Protein Digestion: Protein digestion occurs in the stomach and duodenum in which 3 main enzymes, pepsin secreted by the stomach and trypsin and chymotrypsin secreted by the pancreas, break down food proteins into polypeptides that are then broken down by various exopeptidases and dipeptidases into amino acids. The digestive enzymes however are mostly secreted as their inactive precursors, the zymogens. For example, trypsin is secreted by pancreas in the form of trypsinogen, which is activated in the duodenum by enterokinase to form trypsin. Trypsin then cleaves proteins to smaller polypeptides.

Fat Digestion: Digestion of some fats can begin in the mouth where lingual lipase breaks down some short chain lipids into diglycerides. The presence of fat in the small intestine produces hormones that stimulate the release of pancreatic lipase from the pancreas and bile from the liver for breakdown of fats into fatty acids. Complete digestion of one molecule of fat (a triglyceride) results in 3 fatty acid molecules and one glycerol molecule.

Carbohydrate Digestion: In humans, dietary starches are composed of glucose units arranged in long chains called amylose, a polysaccharide. During digestion, bonds between glucose molecules are broken by salivary and pancreatic amylase, resulting in progressively smaller chains of glucose. This results in simple sugars glucose and maltose (2 glucose molecules) that can be absorbed by the small intestine. Lactase is an enzyme that breaks down the disaccharide lactose to its component parts, glucose and galactose. Glucose and galactose can be absorbed by the small intestine. Approximately half of the adult population produce only small amounts of lactase and are unable to eat milk-based foods. This is commonly known as lactose intolerance. Sucrase is an enzyme that breaks down the disaccharide sucrose, commonly known as table sugar, cane sugar, or beet sugar. Sucrose digestion yields the sugars fructose and glucose which are readily absorbed by the small intestine.

DNA and RNA Digestion: DNA and RNA are broken down into mononucleotides by the nucleases deoxyribonuclease and ribonuclease (DNase and RNase) from the pancreas.

Digestive Hormones

There are at least five hormones that aid and regulate the digestive system in mammals. There are variations across the vertebrates, as for instance in birds. Arrangements are complex and additional details are regularly discovered. For instance, more connections to metabolic control (largely the glucose-insulin system) have been uncovered in recent years.

- Gastrin - is in the stomach and stimulates the gastric glands to secrete pepsinogen (an inactive form of the enzyme pepsin) and hydrochloric acid. Secretion of gastrin is stimulated by food arriving in stomach. The secretion is inhibited by low pH .

- Secretin - is in the duodenum and signals the secretion of sodium bicarbonate in the pancreas and it stimulates the bile secretion in the liver. This hormone responds to the acidity of the chyme.
- Cholecystokinin (CCK) - is in the duodenum and stimulates the release of digestive enzymes in the pancreas and stimulates the emptying of bile in the gall bladder. This hormone is secreted in response to fat in chyme.
- Gastric inhibitory peptide (GIP) - is in the duodenum and decreases the stomach churning in turn slowing the emptying in the stomach. Another function is to induce insulin secretion.
- Motilin - is in the duodenum and increases the migrating myoelectric complex component of gastrointestinal motility and stimulates the production of pepsin.

Significance of pH in Digestion

Digestion is a complex process controlled by several factors. pH plays a crucial role in a normally functioning digestive tract. In the mouth, pharynx, and esophagus, pH is typically about 6.8, very weakly acidic. Saliva controls pH in this region of the digestive tract. Salivary amylase is contained in saliva and starts the breakdown of carbohydrates into monosaccharides. Most digestive enzymes are sensitive to pH and will denature in a high or low pH environment. The stomach's high acidity inhibits the breakdown of carbohydrates within it. This acidity confers two benefits: it denatures proteins for further digestion in the small intestines, and provides non-specific immunity, damaging or eliminating various pathogens.

In the small intestines, the duodenum provides critical pH balancing to activate digestive enzymes. The liver secretes bile into the duodenum to neutralize the acidic conditions from the stomach, and the pancreatic duct empties into the duodenum, adding bicarbonate to neutralize the acidic chyme, thus creating a neutral environment. The mucosal tissue of the small intestines is alkaline with a pH of about 8.5.

Uses of Animal's Internal Organs by Humans

- The stomachs of calves have commonly been used as a source of rennet for making cheese.
- The use of animal gut strings by musicians can be traced back to the third dynasty of Egypt. In the recent past, strings were made out of lamb gut. With the advent of the modern era, musicians have tended to use strings made of silk, or synthetic materials such as nylon or steel. Some instrumentalists, however, still use gut strings in order to evoke the older tone quality. Although such strings were commonly referred to as "catgut" strings, cats were never used as a source for gut strings.
- Sheep gut was the original source for natural gut string used in racquets, such as for tennis. Today, synthetic strings are much more common, but the best gut strings are now made out of cow gut.
- Gut cord has also been used to produce strings for the snares that provide a snare drum's characteristic buzzing timbre. While the modern snare drum almost always uses metal wire rather than gut cord, the North African bendir frame drum still uses gut for this purpose.
- "Natural" sausage hulls (or casings) are made of animal gut, especially hog, beef, and lamb. Similarly, Haggis is traditionally boiled in, and served in, a sheep stomach.
- Chitterlings, a kind of food, consist of thoroughly washed pig's gut.
- Animal gut was used to make the cord lines in longcase clocks and for fusee movements in bracket clocks, but may be replaced by metal wire.
- The oldest known condoms, from 1640 AD, were made from animal intestine.

Chapter 6

Hydrozoa: Character and Classification

Hydrozoa (hydrozoans) are a taxonomic class of very small, predatory animals which can be solitary or colonial and which mostly live in saltwater. A few genera within this class live in freshwater.

Hydrozoans are related to jellyfish and corals and belong to the phylum Cnidaria. Some examples of hydrozoans are the Freshwater Jelly (*Craspedacusta sowerbyi*), the freshwater polyps (*Hydra*), *Obelia*, the Portuguese Man o' War (*Physalia physalis*), the chondrophores (Porpitidae), "air fern" (*Sertularia argenta*) and the pink-hearted hydroids (*Tubularia*).

Anatomy

Most hydrozoan species include both a polypoid and a medusoid stage in their life cycle, although there are a number that have only one or the other. For example, *Hydra* has no medusoid stage, while *Liriope* lacks the hydroid stage.

Polyps

The hydroid form is usually colonial, with multiple polyps connected by tubelike *hydrocauli*. The hollow cavity in the middle of the polyp extends into the associated hydrocaulus, so that all the individuals of the colony are intimately connected. Where the hydrocaulus runs along the substrate it form a horizontal root-like stolon that anchors the colony to the ground.

The colonies are generally small, no more than a few centimetres across, and may have a tree-like or fan-like appearance, depending on species. The polyps themselves are usually tiny, although some non-colonial species are much larger, reaching 6 to 9 centimetres (2.4 to 3.5 in), or, in the case of the deep sea *Branchiocerianthus*, a remarkable 2 metres (6.6 ft). The hydrocaulus is usually surrounded by a sheath of chitin and proteins called the *perisarc*. In some species, this extends upwards to also enclose part of the polyps, in some cases including a closable lid through which the polyp may extend its tentacles. In any given colony, the majority of polyps are specialised for feeding.

These have a more or less cylindrical body with a terminal mouth on a raised protuberance called the hypostome, surrounded by a number of tentacles. The polyp contains a central cavity, in which initial digestion takes place. Partially digested food may then be passed into the hydrocaulus for distribution around the colony and completion of the digestion process. Unlike some other cnidarian groups, the lining of the central cavity lacks stinging nematocysts, which are found only on the tentacles and outer surface.

All colonial hydrozoans also include some polyps specialised for reproduction. These lack tentacles and contain numerous buds from which the medusoid stage of the life-cycle is produced. The arrangement and type of these reproductive polyps varies considerably between different groups. In addition to these two basic types of polyp, a few colonial species have other specialised forms. In some, defensive polyps are found, armed with large numbers of stinging cells. In others, one polyp may develop as a large float, from which the other polyps hang down, allowing the colony to drift in open water instead of being anchored to a solid surface.

Medusae

The medusae of hydrozoans are smaller than those of typical jellyfish, ranging from 0.5 to 6 centimetres (0.20 to 2.4 in) in diametre. Although most hydrozoans have a medusoid stage, this is not always free-living, and in many species, exists solely as a sexually reproducing bud on the surface of the hydroid colony. Sometimes these medusoid buds may be so degenerate as to entirely lack tentacles or mouths, essentially consisting of an isolated gonad. The body consists of a dome-like umbrella ringed by tentacles. A tube-like structure hangs down from the centre of the umbrella, and includes the mouth at its tip. Most hydrozoan medusae have just four tentacles, although a number of exceptions exist. Stinging cells are found on the tentacles and around the mouth. The mouth leads into a central stomach cavity. Four radial canals connect the stomach to an, additional, circular canal running around the base of the bell, just above the tentacles. Striated muscle fibres also line the rim of the bell, allowing the animal to move along by alternately contracting and relaxing its body. An additional shelf of tissue lies just inside the rim, narrowing the aperture at the base of the umbrella, and thereby increasing the force of the expelled jet of water.

The nervous system is unusually advanced for cnidarians, or even than in the polyps of the same species. Two nerve rings lie close to the margin of the bell, and send fibres into the muscles and tentacles. The genus *Sarsia* has even been reported to possess organised ganglia. Numerous sense organs are closely associated with the nerve rings. Mostly these are simple sensory nerve endings, but they also include statocysts and primitive light-sensitive ocelli.

Life Cycle

Hydroid colonies are usually dioecious, which means that they have separate sexes - all the polyps in each colony are either male or female, but not usually both sexes in the same colony. In some species, the reproductive polyps, known as gonozooids (or "gonotheca" in thecate hydrozoans) bud off asexually-produced medusae. These tiny, new medusae (which are either male or female) mature and spawn, releasing gametes freely into the sea in most cases. Zygotes become free-swimming planula larvae or actinula larvae that either settle on a suitable substrate (in the case of planulae), or swim and develop into another medusae or polyp directly (actinulae). Colonial hydrozoans include siphonophore colonies, *Hydractinia*, *Obelia*, and many others.

The medusa stage, if present, is the sexually-reproductive life cycle phase (that is, in hydrozoan species that have both polyp and medusa generations). Medusae of these species of Hydrozoa are known as "hydromedusae". Most hydromedusae have shorter life spans than the larger scyphozoan jellyfish. Some species of hydromedusae release gametes shortly after they are themselves released from the hydroids (as in the case of fire corals), living only a few hours, while other species of hydromedusae grow and feed in the plankton for months, spawning daily for many days before their supply of food or other water conditions deteriorate and cause their demise.

Systematics

Hydrozoan systematics is highly complex. Several approaches for expressing their interrelationships were proposed and heavily contested since the late 19th century, but in more recent times a consensus seems to be emerging.

Historically, the hydrozoans were divided into a number of orders, according to their mode of growth and reproduction. Most famous among these was probably the assemblage called "Hydroida", but this group is apparently paraphyletic, united by plesiomorphic (ancestral) traits. Other such orders were the Anthoathecatae, Actinulidae, Laingiomedusae, Polypodiozoa, Siphonophora and Trachylina.

As far as can be told from the molecular and morphological data at hand, the Siphonophora for example were just highly specialised "hydroids," whereas the Limnomedusae - presumed to be a "hydroid" suborder - were simply very primitive hydrozoans and not closely related to the other "hydroids." Therefore, today the hydrozoans are at least tentatively divided into two subclasses, the Leptolinae (containing the bulk of the former "Hydroida" and the Siphonophora) and the Trachylinae, containing the others (including the Limnomedusae). The monophyly of several of the presumed orders in each subclass is still in need of verification. In any case, according to this classification, the hydrozoans can be subdivided as follows, with taxon names emended to end in "-ae":

Class Hydrozoa

- Subclass Leptolinae
    - Order Anthomedusae (= Anthoathecata(e), Athecata(e), Stylasterina(e)) - includes Laingoimedusae but monophyly requires verification

    - o Order Leptomedusae (= Leptothecata(e), Thecaphora(e), Thecata(e))
    - o Order Siphonophorae
- Subclass Trachylinae
    - o Order Actinulidae
    - o Order Limnomedusae - monophyly requires verification; tentatively placed here
    - o Order Narcomedusae
    - o Order Trachymedusae - monophyly requires verification

ITIS uses the same system but unlike here does not use the oldest available names for many groups. In addition, there exists a weird cnidarian parasite, *Polypodium hydriforme*, which lives inside its host's cells. It is sometimes placed in the Hydrozoa, but actually its relationships are better treated as unresolved for the time being - a somewhat controversial 18S rRNA sequence analysis found it to be closer to Myxozoa. It was traditionally placed in its own class Polypodiozoa and this view is presently often seen to reflect the uncertainties surrounding this highly distinct animal.

Hydra, *a Freshwater Genus*

The most widely-known and researched freshwater hydrozoan is Hydra, which is found in slow-moving waters. Hydra has a pedal disc composed of gland cells that helps it attach to substrates, and like all cnidarians uses nematocysts, or "stinging cells," to disable its prey. Hydra eat small crustaceans (such as brine shrimp), insect larvae, and annelid worms. Hydra may reproduce sexually, through the spawning of sperm (and thus insemination of eggs on the female body column), or through asexual reproduction (budding).

Scyphozoa

Scyphozoa is a class within the phylum Cnidaria, sometimes referred to as the "true jellyfish". The class name *Scyphozoa* comes from the Greek word *skyphos* (óêýöïò), denoting a kind of drinking cup and alluding to the cup shape of the organism. Scyphozoans range in geological time from the Ediacaran period through the Recent.

Anatomy

Scyphozoans usually display a four-part symmetry and have an internal gelatinous material called mesoglea, which provides the same structural integrity as a skeleton. The mesoglea includes mobile amoeboid cells originating from the epidermis. Scyphozoans have no durable hard parts, including no head, no skeleton and no specialised organs for respiration or excretion. Marine jellyfish can consist of as much as 99% water and therefore are rarely found in fossil form. Unlike the hydrozoan jellyfish, hydromedusae, scyphomedusae lack a velum, which is a circular membrane beneath the umbrella that helps propels the (usually smaller) hydromedusae through the water. However, a ring of muscle fibres is present within the mesoglea around the rim of the dome, and the jellyfish swims by alternately contracting and relaxing these muscles. The periodic contracting and relaxing propels the jellyfish through the water, allowing it to escape predation or catch its prey.

The mouth opens into a central stomach, from which four interconnected diverticula radiate outwards. In many species, this is further elaborated by a system of radial canals, with or without an additional ring canal towards the edge of the dome. Some genera, such as *Cassiopea*, even have additional, smaller mouths in the oral arms. The lining of the digestive system includes further stinging nematocysts, along with cells that secrete digestive enzymes.

The nervous system usually consists of a distributed net of cells, although some species possess more organised nerve rings. In species lacking nerve rings, the nerve cells are instead concentrated into small structures called *rhopallia*. There are between four and sixteen of these small lobes arranged around the rim of the umbrella, where they coordinate the muscular action allowing the animal to move. Each rhopallium is typically associated with a pair of sensory pits, a statocyst, and sometimes a pigment-cup ocellus.

Reproduction

Most species appear to be gonochorists, with separate male and female individuals. The gonads are located in the stomach lining, and the mature gametes are expelled through the mouth. After fertilization, some species brood their young in pouches on the oral arms, but they are more commonally planktonic. The fertilized egg produces a planula larva which, in most species, quickly attaches itself to the sea bottom. The larva develops into the hydroid stage of the life-cycle, a tiny sessile polyp called a *scyphistoma*. The scyphistoma reproduces asexually, producing similar polyps by budding, and then either transforming into a medusa, or budding several medusae off from its upper surface. The medusae are initially microscopic, and may take years to reach sexual maturity.

Commercial Importance

Scyphozoa includes the moon jelly *Aurelia aurita*, in the order Semaeostomeae, and the enormous *Nemopilema nomurai*, in the Order Rhizosomeae, found between Japan and China and which in some years causes major fisheries disruptions. Most of the jellyfish that are fished commercially for food are scyphomedusae in the order Rhizostomeae. Most rhizostome jellyfish live in warm water.

In Popular Culture

Scyphozoa is the name of a fictional monster in the animated series *Code Lyoko*.

Anthozoa

Anthozoa is a class within the phylum Cnidaria that contains the sea anemones and corals. Unlike other cnidarians, anthozoans do not have a medusa stage in their development. Instead, they release sperm and eggs that form a planula, which attaches to some substrate on which the cnidarian grows. Some anthozoans can also reproduce asexually through budding. More than 6,100 species have been described. The name comes from the Greek words Üíèïò (*ánthos*; "flower") and æþá (*zóa*; "animals"), hence *anthozoa* = "flower animals", a reference to the floral appearance of their perennial polyp stage.

Biology and Anatomy

Like those of other cnidarians, the individual polyps have a cylindrical body crowned by a ring of tentacles surrounding the mouth. The mouth leads into a tubular pharynx which descends for some distance into the body before opening into the gastrovascular cavity that fills the interior of the body and tentacles. Unlike other cnidarians, however, the cavity is subdivided by a number of radiating partitions, or mesenteries. The gonads are also located within the cavity walls. All cnidarian species can feed by catching prey with nematocysts; sea anemones are capable of catching fish and corals of catching plankton. Some of the species also harbour a type of algae, dinoflagellates called zooxanthellae, in a symbiotic relationship; the reef building corals known as hermatypic corals rely on this symbiotic relationship particularly.

The zooxanthellae benefit by using nitrogenous waste and carbon dioxide produced by the host or , and the cnidarian gains photosynthetic capability and increased calcium carbonate production in hermatypic corals. Anemones and certain species of coral live in isolation, however most corals form colonies of genetically identical polyps; these polyps closely resemble anemonies in structure, although are generally considerably smaller. Most kinds of stony coral live in all parts of the underwater world.

Ctenophora

The Ctenophora are a phylum of animals that live in marine waters worldwide. Their most distinctive feature is the "combs", groups of cilia they use for swimming, and they are the largest animals that swim by means of cilia – adults of various species range from a few millimetres to 1.5 metres (59 in) in size. Like cnidarians, their bodies consist of a mass of jelly, with one layer of cells on the outside and another lining the internal cavity.

In ctenophores, these layers are two cells deep, while those in cnidarians are only one cell deep. Ctenophores also resemble cnidarians in having a decentralized nerve net rather than a brain. Some authors combined ctenophores and cnidarians in one phylum, Coélenterata, as both groups rely on water flow through the body cavity for both digestion and respiration. Increasing awareness of the differences persuaded more recent authors to classify them in separate phyla. Almost all ctenophores are predators, taking prey ranging from microscopic larvae and rotifers to the adults of small crustaceans; the exceptions are juveniles of two species, which live as parasites on the salps on which adults of their species feed. In favourable circumstances, ctenophores can eat ten times their own weight in a day. Only 100–150 species have been validated, and possibly another 25 have not been fully described and named.

The textbook examples are cydippids with egg-shaped bodies and a pair of retractable tentacles fringed with tentilla ("little tentacles") that are covered with colloblasts, sticky cells that capture prey. The phylum has a wide range of body forms, including the flattened, deep-sea platyctenids, in which the adults of most species lack combs, and the coastal beroids, which lack tentacles and prey on other ctenophores by using huge mouths armed with groups of large, stiffened cilia that act as teeth. These variations enable different species to build huge populations in the same area, because they specialise in different types of prey, which they capture by as wide a range of methods as spiders use. Most species are hermaphrodites, in other words a single animal can produce both eggs and sperm; if they are both produced at the same time, the animal is a simultaneous hermaphrodite, and if the eggs and sperm mature at different times, the animal is a sequential hermaphrodite. Fertilization is generally external, although platyctenids' eggs are fertilized inside their parents' bodies and kept there until they hatch.

The young are generally planktonic and in most species look like miniature cydippids, gradually changing into their adult shapes as they grow. The exceptions are the beroids, whose young are miniature beroids with large mouths and no tentacles, and the platyctenids, whose young live as cydippid-like plankton until they reach near-adult size, but then sink to the bottom and rapidly metamorphose into the adult form. In at least some species, juveniles are capable of reproduction before reaching the adult size and shape. The combination of hermaphroditism and early reproduction enables small populations to grow at an explosive rate. Ctenophores may be abundant during the summer months in some coastal locations, but in other places they are uncommon and difficult to find. In bays where they occur in very high numbers, predation by ctenophores may control the populations of small zooplanktonic organisms such as copepods, which might otherwise wipe out the phytoplankton (planktonic plants), which are a vital part of marine food chains. One ctenophore, *Mnemiopsis*, has accidentally been introduced into the Black Sea, where it is blamed for causing fish stocks to collapse by eating both fish larvae and organisms that would otherwise have fed the fish. The situation was aggravated by other factors, such as over-fishing and long-term environmental changes that promoted the growth of the *Mnemiopsis* population. The later accidental introduction of *Beroe* helped to mitigate the problem, as *Beroe* preys on other ctenophores. Despite their soft, gelatinous bodies, fossils thought to represent ctenophores, apparently with no tentacles but many more comb-rows than modern forms, have been found in lagerstätten as far back as the early Cambrian, about 525 million years ago.

The position of the ctenophores in the evolutionary family tree of animals has long been debated, and the majority view at present, based on molecular phylogenetics, is that cnidarians and bilaterians are more closely related to each other than either is to ctenophores. A recent molecular phylogenetics analysis concluded that the common ancestor of all modern ctenophores was cydippid-like, and that all the modern groups appeared relatively recently, probably after the Cretaceous–Paleogene extinction event 65.5 million years ago. Evidence accumulating since the 1980s indicates that the "cydippids" are not monophyletic, in other words do not include all and only the descendants of a single common ancestor, because all the other traditional ctenophore groups are descendants of various cydippids.

Common Features

Body Layers: Like those of cnidarians, (jellyfish, sea anemones, etc.), ctenophores' bodies consist of a relatively thick, jelly-like mesoglea sandwiched between two epithelia, layers of cells bound by inter-cell connections and by a fibrous basement membrane that they secrete.

The epithelia of ctenophores have two layers of cells rather than one, and some of the cells in the upper layer have several cilia per cell. The outer layer of the epidermis (outer skin) consists of: sensory cells; cells that secrete mucus, which protects the body; and interstitial cells, which can transform into other types of cell. In specialised parts of the body the outer layer also contains colloblasts, found along the surface of tentacles and used in capturing prey, or cells bearing multiple large cilia, for locomotion. The inner layer of the epidermis contains a nerve net, and myoepithelial cells that act as muscles.

The internal cavity forms: a mouth that can usually be closed by muscles; a pharynx ("throat"); a wider area in the centre that acts as a stomach; and a system of internal canals. These branch through the mesoglea to the most active parts of the animal: the mouth and pharynx; the roots of the tentacles, if present; all along the underside of each comb row; and four branches round the sensory complex at the far end from the mouth – two of these four branches terminate in anal pores.

The inner surface of the cavity is lined with an epithelium, the gastrodermis. The mouth and pharynx have both cilia and well-developed muscles. In other parts of the canal system, the gastrodermis is different on the sides nearest to and furthest from the organ that it supplies. The nearer side is composed of tall nutritive cells that store nutrients in vacuoles (internal compartments), germ cells that produce eggs or sperm, and photocytes that produce bioluminescence. The side furthest from the organ is covered with ciliated cells that circulate water through the canals, punctuated by ciliary rosettes, pores that are surrounded by double whorls of cilia and connect to the mesoglea.

Feeding, Excretion and Respiration: When prey is swallowed, it is liquefied in the pharynx by enzymes and by muscular contractions of the pharynx. The resulting slurry is wafted through the canal system by the beating of the cilia, and digested by the nutritive cells. The ciliary rosettes in the canals may help to transport nutrients to muscles in the mesoglea.

The anal pores may eject unwanted small particles, but most unwanted matter is regurgitated via the mouth. Little is known about how ctenophores get rid of waste products produced by the cells. The ciliary rosettes in the gastrodermis may help to remove wastes from the mesoglea, and may also help to adjust the animal's buoyancy by pumping water into or out of the mesoglea.

Locomotion: The outer surface bears usually eight comb rows, which are used for swimming. The rows are oriented to run from near the mouth (the "oral pole") to the opposite end (the "aboral pole"), and are spaced more or less evenly around the body, although spacing patterns vary by species and in most species the comb rows extend only part of the distance from the aboral pole towards the mouth. The "combs" (also called "ctenes" or "comb plates") run across each row, and each consists of thousands of unusually long cilia, up to 2 millimetres (0.079 in). These normally beat so that the propulsion stroke is away from the mouth, although they can also reverse direction. Hence ctenophores usually swim in the direction in which the mouth is pointing, unlike jellyfish. When trying to escape predators, one species can accelerate to six times its normal speed; some other species reverse direction as part of their escape behaviour, by reversing the power stroke of the comb plate cilia. It is uncertain how ctenophores control their buoyancy, but experiments have shown that some species rely on osmotic pressure to adapt to water of different densities. Their body fluids are normally as concentrated as seawater. If they enter less dense brackish water, the ciliary rosettes in the body cavity may pump this into the mesoglea to increase its bulk and decrease its density, to avoid sinking. Conversely if they move from brackish to full-strength seawater, the rosettes may pump water out of the mesoglea to reduce its volume and increase its density.

Nervous System and Senses: Ctenophores have no brain or central nervous system, but instead have a nerve net (rather like a cobweb) that forms a ring round the mouth and is densest near structures such as the comb rows, pharynx, tentacles (if present) and the sensory complex furthest from the mouth. The largest single sensory feature is the aboral organ (at the opposite end from the mouth). Its main component is a statocyst, a balance sensor consisting of a statolith, a solid particle supported on four bundles of cilia, called "balancers", that sense its orientation. The statocyst is protected by a transparent dome made of long, immobile cilia. A ctenophore does not automatically try to keep the statolith resting equally on all the balancers. Instead its response is determined by the animal's "mood", in other words the overall state of the nervous system. For example if a ctenophore with trailing tentacles captures prey, it will often put some comb rows into reverse, spinning the mouth towards the prey.

Cydippids

Cydippid ctenophores have bodies that are more or less rounded, sometimes nearly spherical and other times more cylindrical or egg-shaped; the common coastal "sea gooseberry," *Pleurobrachia*, sometimes has an egg-shaped body with the mouth at the narrow end, although some individuals are more uniformly round. From opposite sides of the body extends a pair of long, slender tentacles, each housed in a sheath into which it can be withdrawn. Some species of cydippids have bodies that are flattened to various extents, so that they are wider in the plane of the tentacles. The tentacles of cydippid ctenophores are typically fringed with tentilla ("little tentacles"), although a few genera have simple tentacles without these sidebranches. The tentacles and tentilla are densely covered with microscopic colloblasts that capture prey by sticking to it. Colloblasts are specialised mushroom-shaped cells in the outer layer of the epidermis, and have three main components: a domed head with vesicles (chambers) that contain adhesive; a stalk that anchors the cell in the lower layer of the epidermis or in the mesoglea; and a spiral thread that coils round the stalk and is attached to the head and to the root of the stalk. The function of the spiral thread is uncertain, but it may absorb stress when prey tries to escape, and thus prevent the collobast from being torn apart. In addition to colloblasts, members of the genus *Haeckelia*, which feed mainly on jellyfish, incorporate their victims' stinging nematocytes into their own tentacles – some cnidaria-eating nudibranchs similarly incorporate nematocytes into their bodies for defence. The tentilla of *Euplokamis* differ significantly from those of other cydippids: they contain striated muscle, a cell type otherwise unknown in the phylum Ctenophora; and they are coiled when relaxed, while the tentilla of all other known ctenophores elongate when relaxed.

Euplokamis' tentilla have three types of movement that are used in capturing prey: they may flick out very quickly (in 40 to 60 milliseconds); they can wriggle, which may lure prey by behaving like small planktonic worms; and they coil round prey. The unique flicking is an uncoiling movement powered by contraction of the striated muscle. The wriggling motion is produced by smooth muscles, but of a highly specialised type.

Coiling around prey is accomplished largely by the return of the tentilla to their inactive state, but the coils may be tightened by smooth muscle.

There are eight rows of combs that run from near the mouth to the opposite end, and are spaced evenly round the body. The "combs" beat in a metachronal rhythm rather like that of a Mexican wave. From each balancer in the statocyst a ciliary groove runs out under the dome and then splits to connect with two adjacent comb rows, and in some species runs all the way along the comb rows. This forms a *mechanical* system for transmitting the beat rhythm from the combs to the balancers, via water disturbances created by the cilia.

Lobates

The Lobata have a pair of lobes, which are muscular, cuplike extensions of the body that project beyond the mouth. Their inconspicuous tentacles originate from the corners of the mouth, running in convoluted grooves and spreading out over the inner surface of the lobes (rather than trailing far behind, as in the Cydippida). Between the lobes on either side of the mouth, many species of lobates have four auricles, gelatinous projections edged with cilia that produce water currents that help direct microscopic prey toward the mouth. This combination of structures enables lobates to feed continuously on suspended planktonic prey. Lobates have eight comb-rows, originating at the aboral pole and usually not extending beyond the body to the lobes; in species with (four) auricles, the cilia edging the auricles are extensions of cilia in four of the comb rows. Most lobates are quite passive when moving through the water, using the cilia on their comb rows for propulsion, although *Leucothea* has long and active auricles whose movements also contribute to propulsion.

Members of the lobate genera *Bathocyroe* and *Ocyropsis* can escape from danger by clapping their lobes, so that the jet of expelled water drives them backwards very quickly. Unlike cydippids, the movements of lobates' combs are coordinated by nerves rather than by via water disturbances created by the cilia, yet combs on the same row beat in the same Mexican wave style as the mechanically-coordinated comb rows of cydippids and beroids. This may have enabled lobates to grow larger than cydippids and to have shapes that are less egg-like. An unusual species first described in 2000, *Lobatolampea tetragona*, has been classified as a lobate, although the lobes are "primitive" and the body is medusa-like when floating and disk-like when resting on the sea-bed.

Beroids

The Beroida, also known as Nuda, have no feeding appendages, but their large pharynx, just inside the large mouth and filling most of the saclike body, bears "macrocilia" at the oral end. These fused bundles of several thousand large cilia are able to "bite" off pieces of prey that is too large to swallow whole – almost always other ctenophores. In front of the field of macrocilia, on the mouth "lips" in some species of *Beroe*, is a pair of narrow strips of adhesive epithelial cells on the stomach wall that "zip" the mouth shut when the animal is not feeding, by forming intercellular connections with the opposite adhesive strip. This tight closure streamlines the front of the animal when it is pursuing prey.

Other Body Forms

The Ganeshida have a pair of small oral lobes and a pair of tentacles. The body is circular rather than oval in cross-section, and the pharynx extends over the inner surfaces of the lobes. The Thalassocalycida, only discovered in 1978 and known from only one species, are medusa-like, with bodies that are shortened in the oral-aboral direction, and short comb-rows on the surface furthest from the mouth, originating from near the aboral pole. They capture prey by movements of the bell and possibly by using two short tentacles. The Cestida ("belt animals") are ribbon-shaped planktonic animals, with the mouth and aboral organ aligned in the middle of opposite edges of the ribbon. There is a pair of comb-rows along each aboral edge, and tentilla emerging from a groove all along the oral edge, which stream back across most of the wing-like body surface. Cestids can swim by undulating their bodies as well as by the beating of their comb-rows. There are two known species, with worldwide distribution in warm, and warm-temperate waters: *Cestum veneris* ("Venus' girdle") is among the largest ctenophores – up to 1.5 metres (4.9 ft) long, and can undulate slowly or quite rapidly. *Velamen parallelum*, which is typically less than 20 centimetres (0.66 ft) long, can move much faster in what has been described as a "darting motion".

Most Platyctenida have oval bodies that are flattened in the oral-aboral direction, with a pair of tentilla-bearing tentacles on the aboral surface. They cling to and creep on surfaces by everting the pharynx and using it as a muscular "foot". All but one of the known platyctenid species lack comb-rows. Platyctenids are usually cryptically-coloured, live on rocks, algae, or the body surfaces of other invertebrates, and are often revealed by their long tentacles with many sidebranches, seen streaming off the back of the ctenophore into the current.

Evolutionary History

Fossil Record

Because of their soft, gelatinous bodies, ctenophores are extremely rare as fossils, and fossils that have been interpreted as ctenophores have been found only in lagerstätten, places where the environment was exceptionally suited to preservation of soft tissue. Until the mid-1990s only two specimens good enough for analysis were known, both from the early Devonian period.

Three additional putative species were then found in the Burgess Shale and other Canadian rocks of similar age, about 505 million years ago in the mid-Cambrian period. All three apparently lacked tentacles but had between 24 and 80 comb rows, far more than the 8 typical of living species. They also appear to have had internal organ-like structures unlike anything found in living ctenophores.

One of the fossil species first reported in 1996 had a large mouth, apparently surrounded by a folded edge that may have been muscular. Evidence from China a year later suggests that such ctenophores were widespread in the Cambrian, but perhaps very different from modern species – for example one fossil's comb-rows were mounted on prominent vanes.

The early Cambrian sessile frond-like fossil *Stromatoveris*, from China's Chengjiang lagerstätte and dated to about 525 million years ago, is very similar to Vendobionta of the preceding Ediacaran period. De-Gan Shu, Simon Conway Morris *et al.* found on its branches what they considered rows of cilia, used for filter feeding. They suggested that *Stromatoveris* was an evolutionary "aunt" of ctenophores, and that ctenophores originated from sessile animals whose descendants became swimmers and changed the cilia from a feeding mechanism to a propulsion system.

Relationship to Other Animal Phyla

The position of Ctenophora in the family tree of animals has been debated for many years and is still unclear. Ctenophores have been purported to be the sister lineage to the Bilateria , sister to the Cnidaria, sister to Cnidaria, Placozoa and Bilateria , and sister to all other animal phyla. Recent genomic evidence based on presence and absence of homeoboxes suggests that ctenophores are either sister to Cnidaria, Placozoa and Bilateria or sister to all other animal phyla. The relationship of ctenophores to the rest of the Metazoa is still an open question and is very important to our understanding of the early evolution of animal complexity and the origin of multicellularity.

Relationships within Ctenophora

Since all modern ctenophores except the beroids have cydippid-like larvae, it has widely been assumed that their last common ancestor also resembled cydippids, having an egg-shaped body and a pair of retractable tentacles. Richard Harbison's purely morphological analysis in 1985 concluded that the cydippids are not monophyletic, in other words do not contain all and only the descendants of a single common ancestor that was itself a cydippid. Instead he found that various cydippid families were more similar to members of other ctenophore orders than to other cydippids. He also suggested that the last common ancestor of modern ctenophores was either cydippid-like or beroid-like. A molecular phylogeny analysis in 2001, using 26 species including 4 recently-discovered ones, concluded that the cydippids are not monophyletic and that the last common ancestor of modern ctenophores was cydippid-like. It also found that the genetic differences between these species were very small – so small that the relationships between the Lobata, Cestida and Thalassocalycida remained uncertain.

This suggests that the last common ancestor of modern ctenophores was relatively recent, and perhaps was lucky enough to survive the Cretaceous–Paleogene extinction event

65.5 million years ago while other lineages perished. When the analysis was broadened to include representatives of other phlya, it concluded that cnidarians are probably more closely related to bilaterians than either group is to ctenophores but that this diagnosis is uncertain.

Tentaculata

Tentaculata is a class of comb jellies. The common feature of this class is a pair of long, feathery, contractile tentacles, which can be retracted into specialised ciliated sheaths. In some species, the primary tentacles are reduced and they have smaller, secondary tentacles. The tentacles have colloblasts, which are sticky-tipped cells that trap small prey. Body size and shape varies widely. The group includes the small, oval sea gooseberries (genus *Pleurobrachia*), found on both Atlantic and Pacific coasts. The more flattened species of the genus *Mnemiopsis*, about 4 inches long (10 cm), are common on the upper Atlantic coast; it has a large mouth and mainly feeds on larval molluscs and cope pods. This species is brilliantly luminescent. The similar, but larger, genus *Leucothea* is abundant on the Pacific coast. Venus' girdle (genus *Cestum*) is a flattened, ribbon-like form reaching over 3 feet (90 cm) in length, and found in tropical waters.

Nuda

Nuda is a class of ctenophores or comb jellies. The class contains a single family, Beroidae, with two genera, *Beroe* and *Neis*, and the group is more commonly referred to as the "beroids". They are distinguished from other comb jellies by the complete absence of tentacles, in both juvenile and adult stages. *Beroe* is found in all the world's oceans and seas, and the monotypic *Neis* occurs only near Australia; all beroids are free-swimmers in the plankton.

Anatomy

Some members of the diverse genus *Beroe* may occasionally attain a length of up to 30 centimetres (12 in), though most species and individuals are less than about 10 cm; *Neis cordigera* is among largest species in the class. The sack-like body of the *Beröe* species may be cylindrical in cross section, or compressed to varying amounts by species, while *Neis* is somewhat flattened and characterised by a pair of trailing gelatinous "wings"that extend beyond the aboral pole. Like other comb jellies, the body wall of nudans consists of an outer epidermis and an inner gastrodermis, separated by a jelly-like mesoglea. The mesoglea has pigments that give many nudan species a slightly pink colour; *Neis cordigera* may be yellowish or a deep orange-red.

Mouth Opening and Muscles

Nudans have a very large oral cavity, allowing them to swallow prey whole. While swimming, and particularly while pursuing prey, it can close this mouth like a zipper so that the nuda maintains a streamlined profile. The nuda "zips" its mouth closed from each end, and the "lips" seal shut by forming temporary inter-cellular connections. The whole ctenophore nerve network is within the "lip" of the Nuda of about 40 nerve cell Fort records (Neurit), this bundle of compacted. The palate is caused by the interplay of three different types of muscle open and closed: In the mesoglea lost both ring around the longitudinal axis of the animal and arranged radial, radially outwards from the inside running muscle fibres; they interact with longitudinal, so längsseitig oriented fibres, which the epidermis. Nudans have only smooth muscle fibres.

Macrocilia

Directly inside the mouth opening can be found in the lining of the gap characteristic finger-like excesses, *Macrocilia.* In this first 1844 of JGF Will described and 1965 by George Adrian Horridge with her today named structures are conical shaped by a common plasma membrane surrounded bundles of two to three scourges (cilia), which, as in the comb plates of ribs to a functional unit connected. The individual, between 35 and 60 micrometres in diametre long and 5 to 10 micrometres thick cilia together in a hexagonal cross-sectional structure, and are perpendicular to the direction of common connected by crossbars, a separate membrane, which they divide their neighbour scourges would have it they are not. Each cilium shows the typical eukaryote construction of nine external and two internal microtubules. The scourge cells, in which the cilia from individual basal bodies arise, to the Schlundauskleidung by an average of thirty degrees to mundabgewandten side and, stacked on top like roof tiles. Thus, the macrocilia always point in the direction of the interior of the throat. This is where is the effective strike, which is prey parts in synchronized waves like a conveyor belt transported in the stomach and the throat muscles promoted this process. Macrocilia run in a three toothed top of this is stiff enough to the soft outer wall to rip even larger prey like other ctenophores; proteolytic enzyme penetrate into the resulting wounds, make the victim then quickly escape. Macrocilia also function as teeth, and can be used in the same way as the tentacles of Tentaculata.

Affairs Channel System

From the main drag from stomach like all ctenophore channels in all regions of the body. Each rib will comb through its own meridional canal furnished directly below this location. He owns at the Nuda species many fine ramified excesses, some of which deal with the gap unite, but others end up blind. To that end mouth running the meridional canal in a circle around the mouth lying ring channel.

Statocyste and Polepieces

As with all ctenophores, is at the mundabgewandten side Gleichwichtsorgan, statocyst, including the clock for the ribs arranged on the ridge platelets determine. The shock pulse, unlike in the Lobata, is not through the ridge between platelets oblique scourge forwarded tapes, but the fact that the individual comb platelets in turn fall, like dominoes, the subsequent platelet influence.

Immediately below the statocyst is an inlet lined with sensory cells, which contains epithelial tissue has to mouth out in two opposite narrow bands scourge continues, in the throat level of ctenophore run and as a polepieces. You call a strike by its water flow on the statocyst shows and are used by the Nuda-Arten at its border with finger excesses, the papillae occupied whose function is still unclear, but probably also sensory perception. Unlike other groups of ctenophores put them to continue their movement almost exclusively comb ribs.

Diet

Nudans feed on free swimming animals with soft bodies, primarily from other ctenophores, certainly larger than they themselves can be. They actively hunt for prey, which they usually devour whole. Some species use their macrocilia as teeth to take smaller chunks from the prey.

As Invasive Species

In the late 1980s the ctenophore species *Mnemiopsis leidyi* was introduced into the Black Sea, probably through ballast water, which led to the collapse of the local anchovy population. In 1997 another ctenophore species arrived—*Beroe ovata*, a predator of *Mnemiopsis leidyi*. The Beroe population underwent an initial explosion, until the numbers of both ctenophores stabilized. Nevertheless, both *Mnemiopsis leidyi* and *Beroe ovata* remain today in the Black Sea. The same phenomenon is occurring at the beginning of the 21st century in the Caspian Sea.

Reproduction

All species reproduce sexually, and have both female and male gonad. Although no detailed figures are available, it is assumed that self-fertilization is the exception among nudans. The fertilized eggs hatch into miniature versions of the adult animal, rather than distinct larval forms. They already lack the tentacles and Tentakelscheiden, otherwise they are similar to the *Cydippea* stadum.

History of the Species

There are no known fossil nudans, so the phylogenetic evolution of the group from the comparison with other modern representatives of Rippenquallen tapped to be. In the traditional system, the Nuda form a class distinct from the Tentaculata, which all have at least rudimentary tentacles. This division, after provisional results of morphological and molecular studies, however, probably does not reflect the actual relationships within the ctenophores. Although the scheme is still in the river and does not have an independent assessment of the available evidence, seems to be a family from the order Cydippida, Haeckelidae, in the closer relationship of Nuda species to belong neither Cydippida still Tentaculata would therefore cladistic taxa included not all offspring of their joint Vorfahrens and would therefore is not recognised as a valid taxon in modern schemes. The monophyly of Nuda itself, is however widely accepted, due to the complete lack of tentacles, and the presence of macrocilia as a common secondary feature, or synapomorphy.

Systematics

There are approximately 25 species, grouped into two genera in the single family Beroidae. The family and order were named in 1825 or 1829 by the German naturalist Johann Friedrich Eschscholtz.

- The genus *Beröe* includes nearly all types of class and is distributed worldwide. One of the best known is reflected in the North spread Melonenqualle (*Beröe gracilis*). In *Beröe* species is mundabgewandte (aboral) side down.
- The genus *Neis* is monotypical, containing only one species, *Neis cordigera* (Lesson 1824), and is found only in the waters around Australia. In this type are located on the aboralen page two bogenartige progress rates, so that the middle intermediate aborale Sinnespol unlike the Beroiden not at the extreme end of the body is located (Note Artname *cordigera*: heart). The bogenartigen Fort sentences extend along the flanks of the animal and are Längsverlauf divided so that the impression of two sides "double wings". At the edges of these four "wings" is one rib band. The remaining four ribs on the lost tapes (relative to the "side wings") "upper" and "lower" body half. The ctenophore typical eight ribs number of bands is obtained, even if the tapes because of the particular body shape into two different groups - long training.

Flatworm

The flatworms, known in scientific literature as Platyhelminthes or Plathelminthes (from the Greek ðëáôý, *platy*, meaning "flat" and ëìéíò (root: ëìéíè-), *helminth-*, meaning worm) are a phylum of relatively simple bilaterian, unsegmented, soft-bodied invertebrate animals. Unlike other bilaterians, they have no body cavity, and no specialised circulatory and respiratory organs, which restricts them to flattened shapes that allow oxygen and nutrients to pass through their bodies by diffusion. In traditional zoology texts, Platyhelminthes are divided into Turbellaria, which are mostly nonparasitic animals such as planarians, and three entirely parasitic groups: Cestoda, Trematoda and Monogenea; however, since the turbellarians have since been proven not to be monophyletic, this classification is now deprecated. Free-living flatworms are mostly predators, and live in water or in shaded, humid terrestrial environments such as leaf litter. Cestodes (tapeworms) and trematodes (flukes) have complex life-cycles, with mature stages that live as parasites in the digestive systems of fish or land vertebrates, and intermediate stages that infest secondary hosts.

The eggs of trematodes are excreted from their main hosts, whereas adult cestodes generate vast numbers of hermaphroditic, segment-like proglottids which detach when mature, are excreted, and then release eggs. Unlike the other parasitic groups, the monogeneans are external parasites infesting aquatic animals, and their larvae metamorphose into the adult form after attaching to a suitable host. Because they do not have internal body cavities, for over a century, Platyhelminthes were regarded as a primitive stage in the evolution of bilaterians (animals with bilateral symmetry and hence with distinct front and rear ends). However, analyses since the mid-1980s have separated out one subgroup, the Acoelomorpha, as basal bilaterians - closer to the original bilaterians than to any other modern groups. The remaining Platyhelminthes form a monophyletic group - one that contains all and only descendants of a common ancestor that is itself a member of the group.

The redefined Platyhelminthes is part of the Lophotrochozoa, one of the three main groups of more complex bilaterians. These analyses have also concluded the redefined Platyhelminthes, excluding Acoelomorpha, consists of two monophyletic subgroups, Catenulida and Rhabditophora, and Cestoda, Trematoda and Monogenea form a monophyletic subgroup within one branch of the Rhabditophora. Hence, the traditional platyhelminth subgroup "Turbellaria" is now regarded as paraphyletic, since it excludes the wholly parasitic groups, although these are descended from one group of "turbellarians". Over half of all known flatworm species are parasitic, and some do enormous harm to humans and their livestock. Schistosomiasis, caused by one genus of trematodes, is the second-most devastating of all human diseases caused by parasites, surpassed only by malaria. Neurocysticercosis, which arises when larvae of the pork tapeworm *Taenia solium* penetrate the central nervous system, is the major cause of acquired epilepsy worldwide.

The threat of platyhelminth parasites to humans in developed countries is rising because of organic farming, the popularity of raw or lightly cooked foods, and imports of food from high-risk areas. In less developed countries, people often cannot afford the fuel required to cook food thoroughly, and poorly designed water-supply and irrigation projects increase the dangers presented by poor sanitation and unhygienic farming.

Two planarian species have been used successfully in the Philippines, Indonesia, Hawaii, New Guinea, and Guam to control populations of the imported giant African snail *Achatina fulica*, which was displacing native snails. However, there is now concern that these planarians may themselves become a serious threat to native snails. In northwest Europe, there are concerns about the spread of the New Zealand planarian *Arthurdendyus triangulatus*, which preys on earthworms.

Description

Features Common to All Subgroups

The lack of circulatory and respiratory organs limits platyhelminths to sizes and shapes that enable oxygen to reach and carbon dioxide to leave all parts of their bodies by simple diffusion. Hence, many are microscopic and the large species have flat ribbon-like or leaf-like shapes. The guts of large species have many branches, so nutrients can diffuse to all parts of the body. Respiration through the whole surface of the body makes them vulnerable to fluid loss, and restricts them to environments where dehydration is unlikely: sea and freshwater, moist terrestrial environments such as leaf litter or between grains of soil, and as parasites within other animals.

The space between the skin and gut is filled with mesenchyme, a connective tissue made of cells and reinforced by collagen fibres that act as a type of skeleton, providing attachment points for muscles. The mesenchyme contains all the internal organs and allows the passage of oxygen, nutrients and waste products. It consists of two main types of cell: fixed cells, some of which have fluid-filled vacuoles; and stem cells, which can transform into any other type of cell, and are used in regenerating tissues after injury or asexual reproduction.

Most platyhelminths have no anus and regurgitate undigested material through the mouth. However, some long species have an anus and some with complex, branched guts have more than one anus, since excretion only through the mouth would be difficult for them. The gut is lined with a single layer of endodermal cells which absorb and digest food. Some species break up and soften food first by secreting enzymes in the gut or pharynx (throat). All animals need to keep the concentration of dissolved substances in their body fluids at a fairly constant level.

Internal parasites and free-living marine animals live in environments with high concentrations of dissolved material, and generally let their tissues have the same level of concentration as the environment, while freshwater animals need to prevent their body fluids from becoming too dilute. Despite this difference in environments, most platyhelminths use the same system to control the concentration of their body fluids.

Flame cells, so called because the beating of their flagella looks like a flickering candle flame, extract from the mesenchyme water that contains wastes and some reusable material, and drive it into networks of tube cells which are lined with flagella and microvilli.

The tube cells' flagella drive the water towards exits called nephridiopores, while their microvilli reabsorb reusable materials and as much water as is needed to keep the body fluids at the right concentration. These combinations of flame cells and tube cells are called protonephredia.

In all platyhelminths, the nervous system is concentrated at the head end. This is least marked in the acoels, which have nerve nets rather like those of cnidarians and ctenophores, but densest around the head. Other platyhelminths have rings of ganglia in the head and main nerve trunks running along their bodies.

Major Subgroups

Early classification divided the flatworms into four groups: Turbellaria, Trematoda, Monogenea and Cestoda. This classification had long been recognised to be artificial, and in 1985, Ehlers proposed a phylogenetically more correct classification, where the massively polyphyletic "Turbellaria" was split into a dozen orders, and Trematoda, Monogenea and Cestoda were joined in the new order Neodermata. However, the classification presented here is the early, traditional, classification, as it still is the one used everywhere except in scientific articles.

Turbellaria

The Turbellaria are one of the traditional sub-divisions of the phylum Platyhelminthes (flatworms), and include all the sub-groups that are not exclusively parasitic. There are about 4,500 species, which range from 1 mm (0.039 in) to 600 mm (24 in) in length. All the larger forms are flat with ribbon-like or leaf-like shapes, since their lack of respiratory and circulatory systems means that they have to rely on diffusion for internal transport of metabolites. However, many of the smaller forms are round in cross section. Most are predators, and all live in water or in moist terrestrial environments. Most forms reproduce sexually and with few exceptions all are simultaneous hermaphrodites. The Acoelomorpha and the genus *Xenoturbella* were formerly included in the Turbellaria, but are no longer regarded as Platyhelminthes. All the exclusively parasitic Platyhelminthes form a monophyletic group Neodermata, and it is agreed that these are descended from one small sub-group within the free-living Platyhelminthes. Hence the "Turbellaria" as traditionally defined are paraphyletic.

Description

Traditional classifications divide the Platyhelminthes into four groups: Turbellaria and the wholly parasitic Trematoda, Monogenea and Cestoda. In this classification the Turbellaria include the Acoelomorpha (Acoela and Nemertodermatida). The name "Turbellaria" refers to the "whirlpools" of microscopic particles created close the skins of aquatic species by the movement of their cilia.

Features Common to All Platyhelminthes

Platyhelminthes are bilaterally symmetrical animals, in other words their left and right sides are mirror images of each other; this also implies that they have distinct top and bottom surfaces and distinct head and tail ends. Like other bilaterians they have three main cell layers (it is triploblastic), while the radially symmetrical cnidarians and ctenophore have only two cell layers. Unlike most other bilaterians, platyhelminthes have no internal body cavity and are therefore described as acoelomates. They also lack specialised circulatory and respiratory organs. The lack of circulatory and respiratory organs limits platyhelminths to sizes and shapes that enable oxygen to reach and carbon dioxide to leave all parts of their bodies by simple diffusion. Hence many are microscopic and the large species have flat ribbon-like or leaf-like shapes. The guts of large species have many branches, so that nutrients can diffuse to all parts of the body. Respiration through the whole surface of the body makes platyhelminthes vulnerable to fluid loss, and restricts them to environments where dehydration is unlikely: sea and freshwater; moist terrestrial environments such as leaf litter or between grains of soil; and as parasites within other animals. The space between the skin and gut is filled with mesenchyme, a connective tissue that is made of cells and reinforced by collagen fibres that act as a type of skeleton, providing attachment points for muscles. The mesenchyme contains all the internal organs and allows the passage of oxygen, nutrients and waste products. It consists of two main types of cell: fixed cells, some of which have fluid-filled vacuoles; and stem cells, which can transform into any other type of cell, and are used in regenerating tissues after injury or asexual reproduction. Most platyhelminths have no anus and regurgitate undigested material through the mouth. However some long species have an anus and some with complex branched guts have more than one anus, since excretion only through the mouth would be difficult for them. The gut is lined with a single layer of endodermal cells which absorb and digest food.

Some species break up and soften food first by secreting enzymes in the gut or the pharynx (throat). All animals need to keep the concentration of dissolved substances in their body fluids at a fairly constant level. Internal parasites and free-living marine animals live in environments that have high concentrations of dissolved material, and generally let their tissues have the same level of concentration as the environment, while freshwater animals need to prevent their body fluids from becoming too dilute. Despite this difference in environments, most platyhelminths use the same system to control the level of concentration in their body fluids. Flame cells, so called because the beating of their flagella looks like a flickering candle flame, extract from the mesenchyme water that contains wastes and some re-usable material, and drive it into networks of tube cells which are lined with flagella and microvilli. The tube cells' flagella drive the water towards exits called nephridiopores, while their microvilli re-absorb re-usable materials and as much water as is needed to keep the body fluids at the right level of concentration. These combinations of flame cells and tubule cells are called protonephredia. In all platyhelminths the nervous system is concentrated at the head end. Most species have rings of ganglia in the head and main nerve trunks running along their bodies. Planarians are famous for their ability to regenerate if divided by cuts across their bodies. Experiments show that, in fragments that do not already have a head, a new head grows most quickly on those that were closest to the original head. This suggests that the growth of a head is controlled by a chemical whose concentration diminishes from head to tail.

Features Specific to Turbelleria

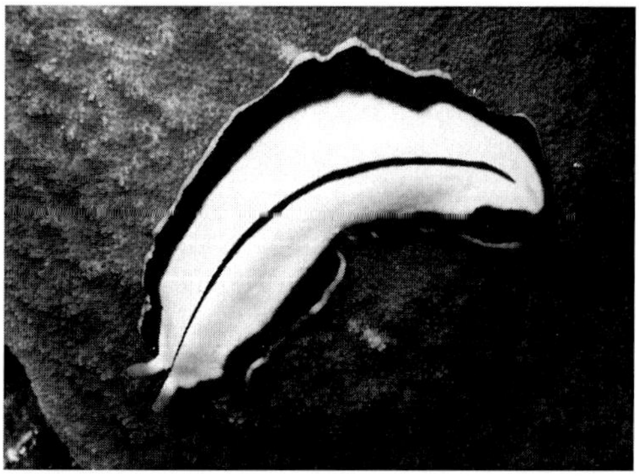

Figure: *The turbellarian Pseudoceros dimidiatus*

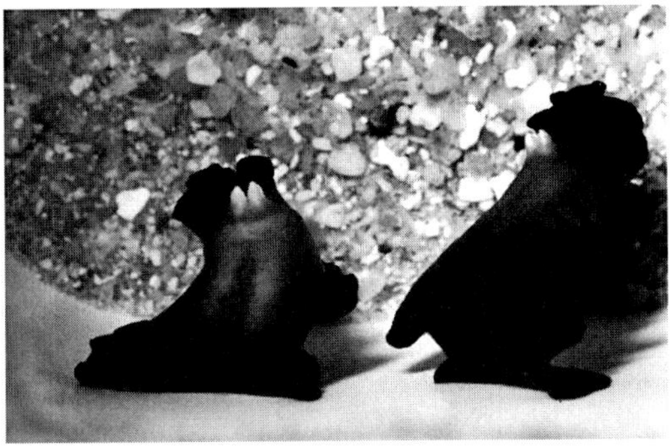

Figure: *Two turbellarians mating by penis fencing. Each has two penises, the white spikes on the undersides of their heads.*

These have about 4,500 species, are mostly free-living, and range from 1 mm (0.039 in) to 600 mm (24 in) in length. Most are predators or scavengers, and terrestrial species are mostly nocturnal and live in shaded humid locations such as leaf litter or rotting wood. However some are symbiotes of other animals such as crustaceans, and some are parasites. Free-living turbellarians are mostly black, brown or gray, but some larger ones are brightly coloured. Turbellarians have no cuticle (external layer of organic but non-cellular material). In a few species the skin is a syncitium, a collection of cells with multiple nuclei and a single shared external membrane. However the skins of most species consist of a single layer of cells, each of which generally has multiple cilia (small mobile "hairs"), although in some large species the upper surface has no cilia. These skins are also covered with microvilli between the cilia. They have many glands, usually submerged in the muscle layers below the skin and connect to the surface by pores through which they secrete mucus, adhesives and other substances.

Small aquatic species use the cilia for locomotion, while larger ones use muscular movements of the whole body or of a specialised sole to creep or swim. Some are capable of burrowing, anchoring their rear ends at the bottom of the burrow, then stretching the head up to feed and then pulling it back down for safety. Some terrestrial species throw a thread of mucus which they use as a rope to climb from one leaf to another. Some Turbelleria have spicular skeletons, giving the appearance of annulations.

Diet and Digestion

The acoel *Convoluta roscoffensis* swallows cells of the green alga *Tetraselmis* and does not feed as an adult, presumably relying on the alge to provide nourishment as endosymbionts. In other acoels the gut is lined by a syncitium. These and some other turbellarians have a simple pharynx lined with cilia and generally feed by using cilia to sweep food particles and small prey into their mouths, which are usually in the middle of the underside. Most other turbellarians are carnivorous, either preying on small invertebrates or protozoans, or scavenging on dead animals. A few feed on larger animals, including oysters and barnacles, while some, such as *Bdelloura*, are commensal on the gills of horseshoe crabs. These turbellarians usually have an eversible pharynx, in other words, one that can be extended by being turned inside-out, and the mouths of different species can be anywhere along the underside. The freshwater species *Microstomum caudatum* can open its mouth almost as wide as its body is long, to swallow prey as large as itself. The intestine is lined by phagocytic cells which capture food particles that have already been partially digested by enzymes in the gut. Digestion is then completed within the phagocytic cells and the nutrients diffuse through the body.

Reproduction

Many turbellarians clone themselves by tranverse or longitudinal division, and others, especially acoels, reproduce by budding. The planarian *Dugesia* is a well-known representative of class Turbellaria. All turbellarians are simultaneous hermaphrodites, having both female and male reproductive cells, and fertilize eggs internally by copulation. Some of the larger aquatic species mate by penis fencing, a duel in which each tries to impregnate the other, and the loser adopts the female role of developing the eggs.

Although the acoels have no distinct gonads at all, in other turbellarians there are one or more pairs of both testes and ovaries. Sperm ducts run from the testes, through bulb-like seminal vesicles, to the muscular penis. In many species, this basic plan is considerably complicated by the addition of accessory glands or other structures. The penis lies inside a cavity, and can be everted through an opening on the posterior underside of the animal. It often, although not always, possesses a sharp stylet. Unusually among animals, in most species, the sperm cells have two tails, rather than one.

In most platyhelminths, the ovaries are divided into two regions, one producing the ova, and the other producing specialised yolk cells to nourish the developing embryo. While many turbellarians have this arrangement, some are apparently more primitive. In these latter species, the ovaries are undivided, and the egg cells contain yolk within their own cytoplasm, as is the case in most other animals. In either arrangement, the ovaries possess oviducts that run to a bursa for storing sperm. The bursa is in turn connected to the vagina, which opens in front of the penis. In some cases, there also be other structures for sperm storage, in addition to the bursa, or even a uterus for storage of ripe eggs. In most species "miniature adults" emerge when the eggs hatch, but a few large species produce plankton-like larvae.

Classification and Evolutionary Relationships

Detailed morphological analyses of anatomical features in the mid-1980s and molecular phylogenetics analyses since 2000 using different sections of DNA agree that Acoelomorpha, consisting of Acoela (traditionally regarded as very simple "turbellarians") and Nemertodermatida (another small group previously classified as "turbellarians") are the sister group to all other bilaterians, including the rest of the "Platyhelminthes".

The "Platyhelminthes" excluding "Acoelomorpha" contain two main groups, Catenulida and Rhabditophora, and it is generally agreed that both are monophyletic, in other words each contains all and only the descendants of an ancestor which is a member of the same group. Early molecular phylogenetics analyses of the Catenulida and Rhabditophora left uncertainties about whether these could be combined in a single monophyletic group, but a study in 2008 concluded that they could, and therefore that "Platyhelminthes" could be redefined as Catenulida plus Rhabditophora, excluding the "Acoelomorpha".

Chapter 7

Sipuncula: Character and Classification

The Sipuncula or Sipunculida (common names sipunculid worms or peanut worms) is a group containing 144-320 species (estimates vary) of bilaterally symmetrical, unsegmented marine worms. Traditionally considered a phylum, molecular work suggests that they might be a subgroup of phylum Annelida.

History

The first species of this phylum was described in 1827 by the French zoologist Henri Marie Ducrotay de Blainville who named it *Sipunculus vulgaris*.

A related species was later described as *Golfingia macintoshii* by E. Ray Lankester.

The specimen was provided by a friend of his Professor Mackintosh. The specimen was dissected by Lankester between rounds of golf at Saint Andrews golf club in Scotland from which the species derives its name. *Golfingia* is now the genus name and *Sipuncula* the name of the phylum to which these worms belong.

Habitat

Sipunculids are all marine and are relatively common, and live in shallow waters, either in burrows or in discarded shells like hermit crabs do.

Some bore into solid rocks to make a shelter for themselves. Although typically less than 10 cm long, some sipunculans may reach several times that length.

Anatomy

Sipunculans are worm-like animals ranging from 2 to 720 millimetres (0.079 to 28 in) in length, with most species being under 10 centimetres (3.9 in). The sipunculan body is divided into an unsegmented trunk and a narrower, retractable anterior section, called the "introvert". Sipunculans have a body wall somewhat similar to that of annelids (though unsegmented) in that it consists of a non-ciliated epidermis overlain by a cuticle, an outer layer of circular and an inner layer of longitudinal musculature. The body wall surrounds the coelom that is filled with fluid on which the body wall musculature acts as a hydrostatic skeleton to extend or contract the animal. When threatened, Sipunculids can retract their body into a shape resembling a peanut kernel - a practice that has given rise to the name "peanut worm". The introvert is retractable into the trunk via two pairs of retractor muscles that extend as narrow ribbons from the trunk wall to attachment points in the introvert. The introvert can be protruded from the trunk by contracting the muscles of the trunk wall, thus forcing the fluid in the body cavity forwards. The sipunculan mouth is located at the anterior end of the introvert, which is surrounded by a mass of 18 - 24 ciliated tentacles in the Sipunculidea. In the Phascolosomatidea, the tentacles are arranged in an arc around the nuchal organ, also located at the tip of the introvert. The tentacles are used to gather organic detritus from the water or substrate, and probably also function as gills. The tentacles at the tip of the introvert are hollow and are extended via hydrostatic pressure in a similar manner as the introvert, but have a separate system from that of the rest of the introvert; they are connected, via a system of ducts, to one or two contractile sacs next to the oesophagus. Hooks are often present near the mouth on the introvert. These are proteinaceous, non-chitinous specialisations of the epidermis which are either arranged in rings or scattered.

Three genera (*Aspidosiphon*, *Lithacrosiphon* and *Cloeosiphon*) possess epidermal modifications, called the anal shield near the anteriorly located anus on the trunk just below the introvert of the animal. In *Aspidosiphon* and *Lithacrosiphon* the anal shield is restricted to the dorsal side, causing the introvert to emerge at an angle, whereas it surrounds the anterior trunk in *Cloeosiphon* with the introvert emerging from its centre. In *Aspidosiphon* the shield is a hardened, horny structure; in *Lithacrosiphon* it is a calcareous cone; in *Cloeosiphon* it is composed of separate plates. At the posterior end, a hardened caudal shield is sometimes present in *Aspidosiphon*.

Digestive System

The digestive tract of Sipunculans starts with the esophagus, located between the introvert retractor muscles. In the trunk the intestine runs posteriorly, forms a loop and turns anteriorly again. The downward and upward sections of the gut are coiled around each other, forming a double helix. At the anterior end of the gut coil the rectum emerges and ends in the anus. A rectal caecum, present in most species, is a blind ending sac at the transition between intestine and rectum with unknown function. The anus is often not visible when the introvert is retracted into the trunk.

Circulation

Sipunclans do not have a vascular blood system. Fluid transport and gas exchange are instead accomplished by the coelom which contains the respiratory pigment haemerythrin, and the tentacular system. The coelomic interstitial fluid contains five types of coelomic cells: haemocytes, granulocytes, large multinuclear cells, ciliated urns and immature cells. The ciliated urn cells may also be attached to the peritoneum and assist in waste filtering from the interstitial fluid. Nitrogenous waste is excreted through a pair of metanephridia opening close to the anus, except in *Phascolion* and *Onchnesoma* which have only a single nephridium. A ciliated funnel, or nephrostome, opens into the coelomic cavity at the anterior end, close to the nephridiopore. The tentacular system connects the tentacles at the tip of the introvert to a ring canal at their base, from which a contractile vessel that runs along the esophagus and ends blindly posteriorly. Some evidence points towards their involvement in ultrafiltration.

Nervous System

The nervous system consists of a nerve ring (the cerebral ganglion) around the oesophagus, which functions as a brain, and a single ventral nerve cord that runs the length of the body.

In some species, there are simple light-sensitive ocelli associated with the brain. Two organs, likely functioning as a unit for chemoreception are located near the anterior margin of the cerebral ganglion: the non-ciliated cerebral organ, which possesses bipolar sensory cells, and the nuchal organ, located posterior to the cerebral organ. In addition, all sipunculans have numerous sensory nerve endings on the body, especially at the forward end of the introvert.

Reproduction

Both asexual and sexual reproduction can be found in Sipunculans, although asexual reproduction is uncommon. Sipunculans reproduce asexually via transverse fission followed by regeneration of vital body components. Most sipunculan species are dioecious. Their gametes are produced in the coelomic lining, where they are released into the coelom to mature. These gametes are then picked up by the metanephridia system and released into the aquatic environment, where fertilisation takes place. Although some species hatch directly into the adult form, many have a trochophore larva, which metamorphoses into the adult after anything from a day to a month, depending on species. In a few species, the trochophore does not develop directly into the adult, but into an intermediate *pelagosphaera* stage, that possesses a greatly enlarged metatroch (ciliated band).

Relationships

The phylogenetic placement of this phylum in the past has proved troublesome. Originally classified as annelids, despite the complete lack of segmentation, bristles and other annelid characters, the phylum Sipuncula was later allied with the Mollusca, mostly on the basis of developmental and larval characters.

Currently these two phyla have been included in a larger group, the Lophotrochozoa, that also includes the annelids, the ribbon worms and several other phyla. Phylogenetic analyses based on 79 ribosomal proteins indicated a position of Sipuncula within Annelida. Subsequent analysis of the mitochondrion's DNA has confirmed their close relationship to the Myzostomida and Annelida (including echiurans and pogonophorans).

Fossil Record

Fossils of sipunculans are extremely rare, and are only known from two genera (*Archaeogolfingia* and *Cambrosipunculus*) from the Cambrian Chengjiang biota in China. These fossils appear to belong to the crown group, and illustrate that sipunculans have changed little since the early Cambrian. Some scientists consider a close relationship of sipunculans and the extinct hyoliths, operculate shells from the Palaeozoic, with which they share the helically twisted gut. If true, the anal plate of some sipunculans might be a remnant of a shell similar to that of hyoliths.

Mollusca

The Mollusca, common name molluscs or mollusks, are a large phylum of invertebrate animals. There are around 85,000 recognised extant species of molluscs. Mollusca is the largest marine phylum, comprising about 23% of all the named marine organisms. Numerous molluscs also live in freshwater and terrestrial habitats. Molluscs are highly diverse, not only in size and in anatomical structure, but also in behaviour and in habitat. The phylum is typically divided into nine or ten taxonomic classes, of which two are entirely extinct. Cephalopod molluscs such as squid, cuttlefish and octopus are among the most neurologically advanced of all invertebrates – and either the giant squid or the colossal squid is the largest known invertebrate species. The gastropods (snails and slugs) are by far the most numerous molluscs in terms of classified species, and account for 80% of the total. Molluscs have such a varied range of body structures that it is difficult to find defining characteristics that apply to all modern groups. The two most universal features are a mantle with a significant cavity used for breathing and excretion, and the structure of the nervous system. As a result of this wide diversity, many textbooks base their descriptions on a hypothetical "generalised mollusc".

This has a single, "limpet-like" shell on top, which is made of proteins and chitin reinforced with calcium carbonate, and is secreted by a mantle that covers the whole upper surface. The underside of the animal consists of a single muscular "foot". Although molluscs are coelomates, the coelom is very small, and the main body cavity is a hemocoel through which blood circulates – molluscs' circulatory systems are mainly open. The "generalised" mollusc's feeding system consists of a rasping "tongue" called a radula and a complex digestive system in which exuded mucus and microscopic, muscle-powered "hairs" called cilia play various important roles. The "generalised mollusc" has two paired nerve cords, or three in bivalves.

The brain, in species that have one, encircles the esophagus. Most molluscs have eyes, and all have sensors that detect chemicals, vibrations and touch. The simplest type of molluscan reproductive system relies on external fertilization, but there are more complex variations. All produce eggs, from which may emerge trochophore larvae, more complex veliger larvae, or miniature adults. A striking feature of molluscs is the use of the same organ for multiple functions.

For example: the heart and nephridia ("kidneys") are important parts of the reproductive system as well as the circulatory and excretory systems; in bivalves, the gills both "breathe" and produce a water current in the mantle cavity, which is important for excretion and reproduction. There is good evidence for the appearance of gastropods, cephalopods and bivalves in the Cambrian period 542 to 488.3 million years ago. However the evolutionary history both of molluscs' emergence from the ancestral Lophotrochozoa and of their diversification into the well-known living and fossil forms are still subjects of vigourous debate among scientists. Molluscs have been and still are an important food source for anatomically modern humans. However there is a risk of food-poisoning from toxins that accumulate in molluscs under certain conditions, and many countries have regulations that aim to minimise this risk. Molluscs have for centuries also been the source of important luxury goods, notably pearls, mother of pearl, Tyrian purple dye, and sea silk. Their shells have also been used as a money in some pre-industrial societies. Mollusc species can also represent hazards or pests for human activities. The bite of the blue-ringed octopus is often fatal, and that of *Octopus apollyon* causes inflammation that can last for over a month. Stings from a few species of large tropical cone shells can also kill, but their sophisticated though easily produced venoms have become important tools in neurological research. Schistosomiasis (also known as bilharzia, bilharziosis or snail fever) is transmitted to humans via water snail hosts, and affects about 200 million people. Snails and slugs can also be serious agricultural pests, and accidental or deliberate introduction of some snail species into new environments has seriously damaged some ecosystems.

Etymology

The words *mollusc* and mollusk are both derived from the French *mollusque*, which originated from the Latin *molluscus*, from *mollis*, soft. *Molluscus* was itself an adaptation of Aristotle's, "the soft things", which he applied to cuttlefish. The scientific study of molluscs is known as malacology. Molluscoida was a name which was formerly used to denote a division of the animal kingdom containing the brachiopods, bryozoans, and tunicates, the members of the three groups having been supposed to somewhat resemble the molluscs. As it is now known that these groups have no relation to molluscs, and very little to one another, the name Molluscoida has been abandoned.

Diversity

Estimates of accepted described living species of molluscs vary from 50,000 to a maximum of 120,000 species. In 2009 Chapman estimated the number of described living species at 85,000. Haszprunar in 2001 estimated about 93,000 named species, which include 23% of all named marine organisms. Molluscs are second only to arthropods in numbers of living animal species—far behind the arthropods' 1,113,000 but well ahead of chordates' 52,000. It has been estimated that there are about 200,000 living species in total, and 70,000 fossil species, although the total number of mollusc species that ever existed, whether or not preserved, must be many times greater than the number alive today. Molluscs have more varied forms than any other animal phylum. They include snails, slugs and other gastropods; clams and other bivalves; squids and other cephalopods; and other lesser-known but similarly distinctive sub-groups. The majority of species still live in the oceans, from the seashores to the abyssal zone, but some form a significant part of the freshwater fauna and the terrestrial ecosystems.

Molluscs are extremely diverse in tropical and temperate regions but can be found at all latitudes. About 80% of all known mollusc species are gastropods. Cephalopoda such as squid, cuttlefish and octopus are among the neurologically most advanced of all invertebrates. The giant squid, which until recently had not been observed alive in its adult form, is one of the largest invertebrates. However a recently caught specimen of the colossal squid, 10 metres (33 ft) long and weighing 500 kilograms (1,100 lb), may have overtaken it.

Freshwater and terrestrial molluscs appear exceptionally vulnerable to extinction. Estimates of the numbers of non-marine molluscs vary widely, partly because many regions have not been thoroughly surveyed. There is also a shortage of specialists who can identify all the animals in any one area to species. However, in 2004 the IUCN Red List of Threatened Species included nearly 2,000 endangered non-marine molluscs. For comparison, the great majority of mollusc species are marine but only 41 of these appeared on the 2004 Red List. 42% of recorded extinctions since the year 1500 are of molluscs, consisting almost entirely of non-marine species.

A "Generalised Mollusc"

Because of the great range of anatomical diversity among molluscs, many textbooks start the subject by describing a hypothetical "generalised mollusc" to illustrate the most common features found within the phylum. The depiction is rather similar to modern monoplacophorans, and some suggest it *may* resemble very early molluscs. The generalised mollusc has a single, "limpet-like" shell on top. The shell is secreted by a mantle that covers the upper surface. The underside consists of a single muscular "foot". The visceral mass, or visceropallium, is the soft, non-muscular metabolic region of the mollusc. It contains the body organs.

Mantle and Mantle Cavity

The mantle cavity is a fold in the mantle that encloses a significant amount of space. It is lined with epidermis. It is exposed, according to habitat, to sea, fresh water or air. The cavity was at the rear in the earliest molluscs but its position now varies from group to group. The anus, a pair of osphradia (chemical sensors) in the incoming "lane", the hindmost pair of gills and the exit openings of the nephridia ("kidneys") and gonads (reproductive organs) are in the mantle cavity. The whole soft body of bivalves lies within an enlarged mantle cavity.

Shell

The mantle edge secretes a shell (secondarily absent in a number of taxonomic groups, such as the nudibranchs) that consists of mainly chitin and conchiolin (a protein) hardened with calcium carbonate), except that the outermost layer in almost all cases is all conchiolin. Molluscs never use phosphate to construct their hard parts, with the questionable exception of *Cobcrephora*. While most mollusc shells are composed mainly of aragonite, those gastropods that lay eggs with a hard shell use calcite (sometimes with traces of aragonite) to construct the eggshells. The shell consists of three layers : the outer layer (the periostracum) made of organic matter, a middle layer made of columnar calcite and an inner layer consisting of laminated calcite, that is often nacreous.

Foot

The underside consists of a muscular foot, which has adapted to different purposes in different classes. The foot carries a pair of statocysts, which act as balance sensors. In gastropods, it secretes mucus as a lubricant to aid movement. In forms that have only a top shell, such as limpets, the foot acts as a sucker attaching the animal to a hard surface, and the vertical muscles clamp the shell down over it; in other molluscs, the vertical muscles pull the foot and other exposed soft parts into the shell. In bivalves, the foot is adapted for burrowing into the sediment; in cephalopods it is used for jet propulsion, and the tentacles and arms are derived from the foot.

Circulation

Molluscs' circulatory systems are mainly open. Although molluscs are coelomates, their coeloms are reduced to fairly small spaces enclosing the heart and gonads. The main body cavity is a hemocoel through which blood and coelomic fluid circulate and which encloses most of the other internal organs. These hemocoelic spaces act as an efficient hydrostatic skeleton. The blood contains the respiratory pigment hemocyanin as an oxygen-carrier. The heart consists of one or more pairs of atria (auricles), which receive oxygenated blood from the gills and pump it to the ventricle, which pumps it into the aorta (main artery), which is fairly short and opens into the hemocoel.

The atria of the heart also function as part of the excretory system by filtering waste products out of the blood and dumping it into the coleom as urine. A pair of nephridia ("little kidneys") to the rear of and connected to the coelom extracts any re-usable materials from the urine and dumps additional waste products into it, and then ejects it via tubes that discharge into the mantle cavity.

Respiration

Most molluscs have only one pair of gills, or even only one gill. Generally the gills are rather like feathers in shape, although some species have gills with filaments on only one side. They divide the mantle cavity so that water enters near the bottom and exits near the top. Their filaments have three kinds of cilia, one of which drives the water current through the mantle cavity, while the other two help to keep the gills clean. If the osphradia detect noxious chemicals or possibly sediment entering the mantle cavity, the gills' cilia may stop beating until the unwelcome intrusions have ceased. Each gill has an incoming blood vessel connected to the hemocoel and an outgoing one to the heart.

Eating, Digestion, and Excretion

Most molluscs have muscular mouths with radulae, "tongues" bearing many rows of chitinous teeth, which are replaced from the rear as they wear out. The radula primarily functions to scrape bacteria and algae off rocks. This radula is associated with the odontophore, a cartilaginous supporting organ. Molluscs mouths also contain glands that secrete slimy mucus, to which the food sticks. Beating cilia (tiny "hairs") drive the mucus towards the stomach, so that the mucus forms a long string. At the tapered rear end of the stomach and projecting slightly into the hindgut is the prostyle, a backward-pointing cone of feces and mucus, which is rotated by further cilia so that it acts as a bobbin, winding the mucus string onto itself. Before the mucus string reaches the prostyle, the acidity of the stomach makes the mucus less sticky and frees particles from it. The particles are sorted by yet another group of cilia, which send the smaller particles, mainly minerals, to the prostyle so that eventually they are excreted, while the larger ones, mainly food, are sent to the stomach's cecum (a pouch with no other exit) to be digested. The sorting process is by no means perfect. Periodically, circular muscles at the hindgut's entrance pinch off and excrete a piece of the prostyle, preventing the prostyle from growing too large. The anus is in the part of the mantle cavity that is swept by the outgoing "lane" of the current created by the gills. Carnivorous molluscs usually have simpler digestive systems. As the head has largely disappeared in bivalves, their mouth has been equipped with labial palps (two on each side of the mouth) to collect the detritus from its mucus.

Nervous System

Molluscs have two pairs of main nerve cords (three in bivalves) the visceral cords serving the internal organs and the pedal ones serving the foot. Both pairs run below the level of the gut, and include ganglia as local control centres in important parts of the body. Most pairs of corresponding ganglia on both sides of the body are linked by commissures (relatively large bundles of nerves). The only ganglia above the gut are the cerebral ganglia, which sit above the esophagus (gullet) and handle "messages" from and to the eyes. The pedal ganglia, which control the foot, are just below the esophagus and their commissure and connections to the cerebral ganglia encircle the esophagus in a nerve ring. The brain, in species that have one, encircles the esophagus. Most molluscs have a head with eyes, and all have a pair of sensor-containing tentacles, also on the head, that detect chemicals, vibrations and touch.

Reproduction

The simplest molluscan reproductive system relies on external fertilization, but there are more complex variations. All produce eggs, from which may emerge trochophore larvae, more complex veliger larvae, or miniature adults. Two gonads sit next to the coelom, a small cavity that surrounds the heart and shed ova or sperm into the coloem, from which the nephridia extract them and emit them into the mantle cavity. Molluscs that use such a system remain of one sex all their lives and rely on external fertilization. Some molluscs use internal fertilization and/or are hermaphrodites, functioning as both sexes; both of these methods require more complex reproductive systems. The most basic molluscan larva is a trochophore, which is planktonic and feeds on floating food particles by using the two bands of cilia round its "equator" to sweep food into the mouth, which uses more cilia to drive them into the stomach, which uses further cilia to expel undigested remains through the anus. New tissue grows in the bands of mesoderm in the interior, so that the apical tuft and anus are pushed further apart as the animal grows. The trochophore stage is often succeeded by a veliger stage in which the prototroch, the "equatorial" band of cilia nearest the apical tuft, develops into the velum ("veil"), a pair of cilia-bearing lobes with which the larva swims. Eventually the larva sinks to the seafloor and metamorphoses into the adult form. Whilst metamorphosis is the usual state in molluscs, the cephalopods differ in exhibiting direct development: the hatchling is a 'miniaturized' form of the adult.

Ecology

Feeding

Most molluscs are herbivorous, grazing on algae. Two feeding strategies are predominant: some feed on microscopic, filamentous algae, often using their radula as a 'rake' to comb up filaments from the sea floor.

Others feed on macroscopic 'plants' such as kelp, rasping the plant itself with its radula. To employ this strategy, the plant has to be large enough for the mollusc to 'sit' on; therefore smaller macroscopic plants enjoy less molluscan herbivory than their larger counterparts. Naturally, there are exceptions; the cephalopods are primarily (perhaps entirely) predatory, and the radula takes a secondary role to the jaws and tentacles in food acquisition.

The monoplacophoran *Neopilina* uses its radula in the usual fashion, but its diet includes protists such as the xenophyophore *Stannophyllum*. Sacoglossan nudibranchs suck the sap from algae, using their one-row radula to pierce the cell walls, whereas dorid nudibranchs and some Vetigastrpods feed on sponges and others feed on hydroids. (An extensive list of molluscs with unusual feeding habits is available in the appendix of GRAHAM, A. (1955). "Molluscan diets". *Journal of Molluscan Studies* 31 (3–4): 144..)

Phylogeny

The phylogeny (evolutionary "family tree") of molluscs is a controversial subject. In addition to the debates about whether *Kimberella* and any of the "halwaxiids" were molluscs or closely related to molluscs, there are debates about the relationships between the classes of living molluscs. In fact some groups traditionally classified as molluscs may have to be redefined as distinct but related. Molluscs are generally regarded members of the Lophotrochozoa, a group defined by having trochophore larvae and, in the case of living Lophophorata, a feeding structure called a lophophore. The other members of the Lophotrochozoa are the annelid worms and seven marine phyla. The diagram on the right summarises a phylogeny presented in 2007.

Because the relationships between the members of the family tree are uncertain, it is difficult to identify the features inherited from the last common ancestor of all molluscs. For example, it is uncertain whether the ancestral mollusc was metameric (composed of repeating units)—if it was, that would suggest an origin from an annelid-like worm. Scientists disagree about this: Giribet and colleagues concluded in 2006 that the repetition of gills and of the foot's retractor muscles were later developments, while in 2007 Sigwart concluded that the ancestral mollusc was metameric, and that it had a foot used for creeping and a "shell" that was mineralized. In one particular one branch of the family tree, the shell of conchiferans is thought to have evolved from the spicules (small spines) of aplacophorans; however this is difficult to reconcile with the embryological origins of spicules. The molluscan shell appears to have originated from a mucus coating, which eventually stiffened into a cuticle. This would have been impermeable and thus forced the development of more sophisticated respiratory apparatus in the form of gills. Eventually, the cuticle would have become mineralized, using the same genetic machinery (*engrailed*) as most other bilaterian skeletons. The first mollusc shell almost certainly was reinforced with the mineral aragonite. The evolutionary relationships *within* the molluscs are also debated, and the diagrams below show two widely supported reconstructions: Morphological analyses tend to recover a conchiferan clade that receives less support from molecular analyses, although these results also lead to unexpected paraphylies, for instance scattering the bivalves throughout all other mollusc groups. However, an analysis in 2009 that used both morphological and molecular phylogenetics comparisons concluded that the molluscs are not monophyletic; in particular, that Scaphopoda and Bivalvia are both separate, monophyletic lineages unrelated to the remaining molluscan classes—in other words that the traditional phylum Mollusca is polyphyletic, and that it can only be made monophyletic if scaphopods and bivalves are excluded. A 2010 analysis managed to recover the traditional conchiferan and aculiferan groups, but similarly concluded that the molluscs are not monophyletic, this time suggesting that solenogastres are more closely related to the non-molluscan taxa used as an outgroup than to other molluscs. Current molecular data is insufficient to constrain the molluscan phylogeny, and since the methods used to determine the confidence in clades are prone to over-estimation, it is risky to place too much emphasis even on the areas that different studies agree. Rather than eliminating unlikely relationships, the latest studies add new permutations of internal molluscan relationships, even bringing the conchiferan hypothesis into question.

Human Interaction

For millennia molluscs have been a source of food for humans, as well as important luxury goods, notably pearls, mother of pearl, Tyrian purple dye, sea silk, and chemical compounds. Their shells have also been used as a form of currency in some pre-industrial societies. Their outlandish forms have helped conjure up tales of mythological sea monsters such as the Kraken. A number of species of molluscs can bite or sting humans, and some have become agricultural pests.

Uses by Humans

Molluscs, especially bivalves such as clams and mussels, have been an important food source since at least the advent of anatomically modern humans—and this has often resulted in over-fishing. Other commonly eaten molluscs include octopuses and squids, whelks, oysters, and scallops. In 2005, China accounted for 80% of the global mollusc catch, netting almost 11,000,000 tonnes (11,000,000 long tons; 12,000,000 short tons). Within Europe, France remained the industry leader. Some countries regulate importation and handling of molluscs and other seafood, mainly to minimise the poison risk from toxins that accumulate in the animals. Most molluscs that have shells can produce pearls, but only the pearls of bivalves and some gastropods whose shells are lined with nacre are valuable. The best natural pearls are produced by marine pearl oysters. *Pinctada margaritifera* and *Pinctada mertensi*, which live in the tropical and sub-tropical waters of the Pacific Ocean. Natural pearls form when a small foreign object gets stuck between the mantle and shell.

There are two methods of culturing pearls, by inserting either "seeds" or beads into oysters. The "seed" method uses grains of ground shell from freshwater mussels, and over-harvesting for this purpose has endangered several freshwater mussel species in the southeastern USA. The pearl industry is so important in some areas that significant sums of money are spent on monitoring the health of farmed molluscs. Other luxury and high-status products were made from molluscs. Tyrian purple, made from the ink glands of murex shells, "... fetched its weight in silver" in the fourth-century BC, according to Theopompus. The discovery of large numbers of Murex shells on Crete suggests that the Minoans may have pioneered the extraction of "Imperial purple" during the Middle Minoan period in the 20th–18th century BC, centuries before the Tyrians.

Sea silk is a fine, rare and valuable fabric produced from the long silky threads (byssus) secreted by several bivalve molluscs, particularly *Pinna nobilis*, to attach themselves to the sea bed. Procopius, writing on the Persian wars circa 550 CE, "stated that the five hereditary satraps (governors) of Armenia who received their insignia from the Roman Emperor were given chlamys (or cloaks) made from *lana pinna* (Pinna "wool," or byssus). Apparently only the ruling classes were allowed to wear these chlamys." Mollusc shells, including those of cowries, were used as a kind of money (shell money) in several pre-industrial societies. However these "currencies" generally differed in important ways from the standardized government-backed and -controlled money familiar to industrial societies. Some shell "currencies" were not used for commercial transactions but mainly as social status displays at important occasions such as weddings. When used for commercial transactions they functioned as commodity money, in other words as a tradable commodity whose value differed from place to place, often as a result of difficulties in transport, and which was vulnerable to incurable inflation if more efficient transport or "goldrush" behaviour appeared.

Stings and Bites

There is a risk of food poisoning from toxins that accumulate in molluscs under certain conditions, and many countries have regulations that aim to minimise this risk. Blue-ringed octopus bites are often fatal, and the bite of other octopuses can cause unpleasant symptoms.

Stings from a few species of large tropical cone shells can also kill. However, the sophisticated venoms of these cone snails have become important tools in neurological research and show promise as sources of new medications. When handled alive, a few species of molluscs can sting or bite and, with some species, this can present a serious risk to the human handling the animal. To put this into perspective however, deaths from mollusc venoms are less than 10% of the number of deaths from jellyfish stings.

All octopuses are venomous but only a few species pose a significant threat to humans. Blue-ringed octopuses in the genus *Hapalochlaena*, which live around Australia and New Guinea, bite humans only if severely provoked, but their venom kills 25% of human victims. Another tropical species, *Octopus apollyon*, causes severe inflammation that can last for over a month even if treated correctly, and the bite of *Octopus rubescens* can cause necrosis that lasts longer than one month if untreated, and headaches and weakness persisting for up to a week even if treated. All species of cone snails are venomous and can sting when handled, although many species are too small to pose much of a risk to humans. These are carnivorous gastropods that feed on marine invertebrates (and in the case of larger species on fish).

Their venom is based on a huge array of toxins, some fast-acting and others slower but deadlier—they can afford to do this because their toxins require less time and energy to be produced compared with those of snakes or spiders. Many painful stings have been reported, and a few fatalities, although some of the reported fatalities may be exaggerations. Only the few larger species of cone snail that can capture and kill fish are likely to be seriously dangerous to humans. The effects of individual cone shell toxins on victims' nervous systems are so precise that they are useful tools for research in neurology, and the small size of their molecules makes it easy to synthesize them. The traditional belief that a giant clam can trap the leg of a person between its valves, thus drowning them, is a myth.

Pests

Schistosomiasis (also known as bilharzia, bilharziosis or snail fever) is transmitted to humans via water snail hosts, and affects about 200 million people. A few species of snails and slugs are serious agricultural pests, and in addition, accidental or deliberate introduction of various snail species into new territory has resulted in serious damage to some natural ecosystems. Schistosomiasis is "second only to malaria as the most devastating parasitic disease in tropical countries. An estimated 200 million people in 74 countries are infected with the disease — 100 million in Africa alone." The parasite has 13 known species, of which two infect humans. The parasite itself is not a mollusc, but all the species have freshwater snails as intermediate hosts.

Some species of molluscs, particularly certain snails and slugs, can be serious crop pests, and when introduced into new environments can unbalance local ecosystems. One such pest, the giant African snail *Achatina fulica*, has been introduced to many parts of Asia, as well as to many islands in the Indian Ocean and Pacific Ocean.

In the 1990s this species reached the West Indies. Attempts to control it by introducing the predatory snail *Euglandina rosea* proved disastrous, as the predator ignored *Achatina fulica* and went on to extirpate several native snail species instead. Despite its name, *Molluscum contagiosum* is a viral disease, and is unrelated to molluscs.

Chiton

Chitons are small to large marine molluscs in the class Polyplacophora, which formerly was known as Amphineura.

There are approximately 940 extant and 430 fossil species recognised. These molluscs are also sometimes commonly known as sea cradles or "coat-of-mail shells". They are also sometimes referred to more formally as loricates, polyplacophorans, and rarely as polyplacophores.

Chitons have a dorsal shell which is composed of eight separate shell plates or valves. These plates overlap somewhat at the front and back edges, and yet the plates articulate well with one another. Because of this, although the plates provide good protection for impacts from above, they nonetheless permit the chiton to flex upward when needed for locomotion over uneven surfaces, and also the animal can slowly curl up into a ball when it is dislodged from the underlying surface. The shell plates are surrounded by a structure known as a girdle.

Habitat

Chitons live worldwide, in cold water, warm water, and in the tropics. Most chiton species inhabit intertidal or sub tidal zones, and do not extend beyond the photic zone. They live on hard surfaces, such as on or under rocks, or in rock crevices. Some species live quite high in the intertidal zone and are exposed to the air and light for long periods. Others live subtidally. A few species live in deep water, as deep as 6,000 metres (20,000 ft). Chitons are exclusively and fully marine. This is in contrast to the bivalves which were able to adapt to brackish water and freshwater, and the gastropods which were able to make successful transitions to freshwater and terrestrial environments.

Morphology

Shell

All chitons bear a row of aragonitic shells, although in some species they are reduced or covered by the girdle tissue. The calcareous valves that chitons carry dorsally are protective, made wholly of aragonite, and variously coloured, patterned, smooth or sculptured. The shell is divided into eight articulating calcareous (aragonite) valves embedded in the tough muscular girdle that surrounds the chiton's body. This arrangement allows chitons to roll into a protective ball when dislodged and to cling tightly to irregular surfaces. The most anterior plate is crescent shaped, and is known as the cephalic plate (sometimes called a "head plate", despite the absence of a complete head). The most posterior plate is known as the anal plate (sometimes called the "tail plate", although chitons do not have a tail.)

The front simultaneously, with the rear plate being added later in the developmental process. Growth lines are formed each winter. The inner layer of each of the six intermediate plates is produced anteriorly as an articulating flange. This is called the *articulamentum*. This inner layer may also be produced laterally in the form of notched *insertion plates*. These function as an attachment of the valve plates to the soft body. A similar series of insertion plates may be attached to the convex anterior border of the cephalic plate or the convex posterior border of the anal plate. The sculpture of the valves is one of the taxonomic characteristics, along with the granulation or spinulation of the girdle After a chiton dies, the individual valves which make up the 8-part shell come apart because the girdle is no longer holding them together, and then the plates sometimes wash up in beach drift. The individual shell plates from a chiton are sometimes known as "butterfly shells" because of their shape.

Girdle Ornament

The girdle may be ornamented with scales or spicules which, like the shell plates, are mineralized with aragonite – although a different mineralization process operates in the spicules to in the teeth or shells (implying an independent evolutionary innovation). This process seems quite simple in comparison to other shelly tissue; the crystal structure of the deposited minerals closely resembles the disordered nature of crystals that form inorganically.

The protein component of the scales and sclerites is minuscule in comparison with other biomineralized structures, whereas the total proportion of matrix is *higher* than in mollusc shells. This implies that polysaccharides make up the bulk of the matrix.

The girdle spines often bear length-parallel striations. The wide form of girdle ornament suggests that it serves a secondary role; chitons can survive perfectly well without them. Camouflage or defence are two likely functions.

Internal Anatomy

The girdle is often ornamented with spicules, bristles, hairy tufts, spikes, or snake-like scales. The majority of the body is a snail-like foot, but no head or other soft-parts beyond the girdle are visible from the dorsal side. The mantle cavity consists of a narrow channel on each side, lying between the body and the girdle. Water enters the cavity through openings either side of the mouth, then flows along the channel to a second, exhalant, opening close to the anus. Multiple gills hang down into the mantle cavity along part or all of the lateral pallial groove, each consisting of a central axis with a number of flattened filaments through which oxygen can be absorbed. The heart has three chambers and is located towards the animal's hind end. Each of the two auricles collects blood from the gills on one side, while the muscular ventricle pumps blood through the aorta and round the body. The excretory system consists of two nephridia, which connect to the pericardial cavity around the heart, and remove excreta through a pore that opens near the rear of the mantle cavity. The single gonad is located in front of the heart, and releases gametes through a pair of pores just in front of those used for excretion. The mouth is located on the underside of the animal, and contains a tongue-like structure called a radula, which has numerous rows of 17 teeth each. The teeth are coated with magnetite, a hard ferric/ferrous oxide mineral.

The radula is used to scrape microscopic algae off the substratum. The mouth cavity itself is lined with chitin and is associated with a pair of salivary glands. Two sacs open from the back of the mouth, one containing the radula, and the other containing a protrusible sensory subradula organ that is pressed against the substratum to taste for food. Cilia pull the food through the mouth in a stream of mucus and through the oesophagus, where it is partially digested by enzymes from a pair of large pharyngeal glands. The oesophagus in turn opens into a stomach with where enzymes from a digestive gland complete the breakdown of the food. Nutrients are absorbed through the linings of the stomach and the first part of the intestine. The intestine is divided in two by a sphincter, with the latter part being highly coiled and functioning to compact the waste matter into faecal pellets. The anus opens just behind the foot. Chitons lack a clearly demarcated head; their nervous system resembles a dispersed ladder. There are no true ganglia as there are in other molluscs, although there is a ring of dense neural tissue around the oesophagus. From this ring, nerves branch forwards to innervate the mouth and subradula, while two pairs of main nerve cords run back through the body. One pair, the pedal cords, innervate the foot, while the pallio-visceral cords innervate the mantle and remaining internal organs. Some species bear an array of tentacles in front of the head.

Senses

The primary sense organs of chitons are the subradula organ and a large number of unique organs called aesthetes. The aesthetes consist of light sensitive cells just below the surface of the shell, although they are not capable of true vision. In some cases, however, they are modified to form ocelli, with a cluster of individual photoreceptor cells lying beneath a small lens. An individual chiton may have thousands of such ocelli. There is a relatively good fossil record of chiton shells, but ocelli are only present in those dating to 10 million years ago or younger; this would make the ocelli, whose precise function is unclear, the most recent eyes to evolve. Although chitons lack osphradia, statocysts, and other sensory organs common to other molluscs, they do have numerous tactile nerve endings, especially on the girdle and within the mantle cavity. However, chitons lack a cerebral ganglion.

Homing Ability

Several species of Chiton are known to exhibit homing behaviours, journeying to feed and then returning to the exact spot they previously inhabited. The method they use to perform such behaviours has been investigated to some extent, but remains unknown. One theory is that the chitons remember the topographic profile of the region, thus being able to guide themselves back to their home scar via a physical knowledge of the rocks and visual input from their numerous primitive eyespots. The sea snail *Nerita textilis* (like all gastropods) deposits a mucus trail as it moves, which a chemoreceptive organ is able to detect and guide the snail back to its home site, It is unclear if chiton homing functions in the same way, but it is theorized that they may leave chemical cues along the rock surface and at the home scar which their olfactory senses can detect and home in on. Furthermore, older trails may also be detected, providing further stimulus for the Chiton to find its home, Chitons have radular teeth made of magnetite (an iron compound) making them unique among animals.

This means they have an exceptionally abrasive tongue with which to scrape algae from rocks. The iron crystals may also be involved in magnetoception, the ability to sense the polarity or the inclination of the Earth's magnetic field, and thus may be used in navigation.

Culinary Uses

Chitons are eaten in many islands in the Caribbean, including Trinidad, Tobago and Barbados. They were also eaten by native Americans of the Pacific coasts of both North and South America. The foot of the chiton is prepared in a manner similar to abalone.

Life Habits

A chiton creeps along slowly on a muscular foot. They have considerable power of adhesion and can cling to rocks very powerfully, like a limpet. Chitons are herbivorous grazers. They eat algae, bryozoans, diatoms and sometimes bacteria by scraping the rocky substrate with their well-developed radula. A few species of chitons are predatory, such as the small western Pacific species *Placiphorella velata*. These predatory chitons have an enlarged anterior girdle. They catch other small invertebrates, such as shrimp and possibly even small fish, by holding the enlarged, hood-like front end of the girdle up off the surface, and then clamping down on unsuspecting, shelter-seeking prey. Some chitons exhibit homing behaviour, returning to the same spot for the daylight hours and roaming around at night to feed.

Reproduction and Life Cycle

Chitons have separate sexes, and fertilization is external. The male releases sperm into the water, while the female releases eggs either individually, or in a long string. In most cases, fertilization takes place either in the surrounding water, or in the mantle cavity of the female. Some species brood the eggs within the mantle cavity, and the species *Callistochiton viviparus* even retains them within the ovary and gives birth to live young, an example of ovoviviparity.

The eggs have a tough spiny coat, and usually hatch to release a free-swimming trochophore larva, typical of many other mollusc groups. In a few cases, the trochophore remains within the egg (and is then called *lecithotrophic* – deriving nutrition from yolk), which hatches to produce a miniature adult.

Unlike most other molluscs, there is no intermediate stage, or veliger, between the trochophore and the adult. Instead, a segmented shell gland forms on one side of the larva, and a foot forms on the opposite side. When the larva is ready to become an adult, the body elongates, and the shell gland secretes the plates of the shell. Unlike the fully grown adult, the larva has a pair of simple eyes, although these may remain for some time in the immature adult.

Predators

Animals which prey on chitons include humans, seagulls, seastars, crabs, lobster and fish.

The Largest Species

The largest chiton (up to 33 cm in length) is the brick-red gumboot chiton of the Pacific Northwest. In this species the valves are completely internal.

History of the Scientific Investigation of Chitons

Chitons were first studied by Carolus Linnaeus in 1758. Since his description of the first four species, chitons have been variously classified. They were called Cyclobranchians ("round arm") in the early 19th century, and then grouped with the aplacophorans in the subphylum Amphineura in 1876. The class Polyplacophora was named by de Blainville 1816.

Etymology

The English name "chiton" originates from the Latin word chitôn, which means "mollusc", and in turn is derived from the Greek word "khitôn", meaning tunic (which also is the source of the word chitin). The Greek word "khitôn" can be traced to the Central Semitic word "*kittan", which is from the Akkadian words "kitû" or "kita'um", meaning flax or linen, and originally the Sumerian word "gada" or "gida". The Greek-derived name Polyplacophora comes from the words poly- (many), plako- (tablet), and -phoros (bearing), a reference to the chiton's eight shell plates.

Taxonomy

Most classification schemes in use today are based, at least in part, on Pilsbry's Manual of Conchology (1892–1894), extended and revised by Kaas and Van Belle (1985–1990). Since chitons were first described by Linnaeus (1758) there have been extensive taxonomic studies at the species level. However, the taxonomic classification at higher levels in the group has remained somewhat unsettled. The most recent classification (Sirenko 2006) is based not only on shell morphology, as usual, but also other important features including aesthetes, girdle, radula, gills, glands, egg hull projections and spermatozoids. It includes all the living and extinct genera of chitons.

This system is now generally accepted.

- Class Polyplacophora de Blainville, 1816
  - o Subclass Paleoloricata Bergenhayn, 1955
    - — Order Chelodida Bergenhayn, 1943
    - — Family Chelodidae Bergenhayn, 1943
    - — *Chelodes* Davidson et King, 1874
    - — *Euchelodes* Marek, 1962
    - — *Calceochiton* Flower, 1968
    - — Order Septemchitonida Bergenhayn, 1955
    - — Family Gotlandochitonidae Bergenhayn, 1955
    - — *Gotlandochiton* Bergenhayn, 1955
    - — Family Helminthochitonidae Van Belle, 1975
    - — *Kindbladochiton* Van Belle, 1975
    - — *Diadelochiton* Hoare, 2000
    - — *Helminthochiton* Salter in Griffith et M'Coy, 1846
    - — *Echinochiton* Pojeta, Eernisse, Hoare et Henderson, 2003
    - — Family Septemchitonidae Bergenhayn, 1955

— *Septemchiton* Bergenhayn, 1955
— *Paleochiton* A. G. Smith, 1964
— *Thairoplax* Cherns, 1998

o Subclass Loricata Shumacher, 1817
— Order Lepidopleurida Thiele, 1910
— Suborder Cymatochitonina Sirenko et Starobogatov, 1977
— Family Acutichitonidae Hoare, Mapes et Atwater, 1983
— *Acutichiton* Hoare, Sturgeon et Hoare, 1972
— *Elachychiton* Hoare, Sturgeon et Hoare, 1972
— *Harpidochiton* Hoare et Cook, 2000
— *Arcochiton* Hoare, Sturgeon et Hoare, 1972
— *Kraterochiton* Hoare, 2000
— *Soleachiton* Hoare, Sturgeon et Hoare, 1972
— *Asketochiton* Hoare et Sabattini, 2000
— Family Cymatochitonidae Sirenko et Starobogatov, 1977
— *Cymatochiton* Dall, 1882
— *Compsochiton* Hoare et Cook, 2000
— Family Gryphochitonidae Pilsbry, 1900
— *Gryphochiton* Gray, 1847
— Family Lekiskochitonidae Smith et Hoare, 1987
— *Lekiskochiton* Hoare et Smith, 1984
— Family Permochitonidae Sirenko et Starobogatov, 1977
— *Permochiton* Iredale et Hull, 1926
— Suborder Lepidopleurina Thiele, 1910
— Family *Abyssochitonidae* (synonym: Ferreiraellidae) Dell' Angelo et Palazzi, 1991
— *Glaphurochiton* Raymond, 1910
— *Pyknochiton* Hoare, 2000
— *Hadrochiton* Hoare, 2000

— *Ferreiraella* Sirenko, 1988
— Family Glyptochitonidae Starobogatov et Sirenko, 1975
— *Glyptochiton* Konninck, 1883
— Family Leptochitonidae Dall, 1889
— *Colapterochiton* Hoare et Mapes, 1985
— *Coryssochiton* DeBrock, Hoare et Mapes, 1984
— *Proleptochiton* Sirenko et Starobogatov, 1977
— *Schematochiton* Hoare, 2002
— *Pterochiton* (Carpenter MS) Dall, 1882
— *Leptochiton* Gray, 1847
— *Parachiton* Thiele, 1909
— *Terenochiton* Iredale, 1914
— *Trachypleura* Jaeckel, 1900
— *Pseudoischnochiton* Ashby, 1930
— *Lepidopleurus* Risso, 1826
— *Hanleyella* Sirenko, 1973
— Family Camptochitonidae Sirenko, 1997
— *Camptochiton* DeBrock, Hoare et Mapes, 1984
— *Pedanochiton* DeBrock, Hoare et Mapes, 1984
— *Euleptochiton* Hoare et Mapes, 1985
— *Pileochiton* DeBrock, Hoare et Mapes, 1984
— *Chauliochiton* Hoare et Smith, 1984
— *Stegochiton* Hoare et Smith, 1984
— Family Nierstraszellidae Sirenko, 1992
— *Nierstraszella* Sirenko, 1992
— Family Mesochitonidae Dell' Angelo et Palazzi, 1989
— *Mesochiton* Van Belle, 1975
— *Pterygochiton* Rochebrune, 1883
— Family Protochitonidae Ashby, 1925
— *Protochiton* Ashby, 1925
— *Deshayesiella* (Carpenter MS) Dall, 1879

— *Oldroydia* Dall, 1894
— Family Hanleyidae Bergenhayn, 1955
— *Hanleya* Gray, 1857
— *Hemiarthrum* Dall, 1876
— Order Chitonida Thiele, 1910
— Suborder Chitonina Thiele, 1910
— Superfamily Chitonoidea Rafinesque, 1815
— Family Ochmazochitonidae Hoare et Smith, 1984
— *Ochmazochiton* Hoare et Smith, 1984
— Family Ischnochitonidae Dall, 1889
— *Ischnochiton* Gray, 1847
— *Stenochiton* H. Adams et Angas, 1864
— *Stenoplax* (Carpenter MS) Dall, 1879
— *Lepidozona* Pilsbry, 1892
— *Stenosemus* Middendorff, 1847
— *Subterenochiton* Iredale et Hull, 1924
— *Thermochiton* Saito et Okutani, 1990
— *Connexochiton* Kaas, 1979
— *Tonicina* Thiele, 1906
— Family Callistoplacidae Pilsbry, 1893
— *Ischnoplax* Dall, 1879
— *Callistochiton* Carpenter MS, Dall, 1879
— *Callistoplax* Dall, 1882
— *Ceratozona* Dall, 1882
— *Calloplax* Thiele, 1909
— Family Chaetopleuridae Plate, 1899
— *Chaetopleura* Shuttleworth, 1853
— *Dinoplax* Carpenter MS, Dall, 1882
— Family Loricidae Iredale et Hull, 1923
— *Lorica* H. et A. Adams, 1852
— *Loricella* Pilsbry, 1893
— *Oochiton* Ashby, 1929

— Family Callochitonidae Plate, 1901
— *Callochiton* Gray, 1847
— *Eudoxochiton* Shuttleworth, 1853
— *Vermichiton* Kaas, 1979
— Family Chitonidae Rafinesque, 1815
— Subfamily Chitoninae Rafinesque, 1815
— *Chiton* Linnaeus, 1758
— *Amaurochiton* Thiele, 1893
— *Radsia* Gray, 1847
— *Sypharochiton* Thiele, 1893
— *Nodiplax* Beu, 1967
— *Rhyssoplax* Thiele, 1893
— *Teguloaplax* Iredale & Hull, 1926
— *Mucrosquama* Iredale, 1893
— Subfamily Toniciinae Pilsbry, 1893
— *Tonicia* Gray, 1847
— *Onithochiton* Gray, 1847
— Subfamily Acanthopleurinae Dall, 1889
— *Acanthopleura* Guilding, 1829
— *Liolophura* Pilsbry, 1893
— *Enoplochiton* Gray, 1847
— *Squamopleura* Nierstrasz, 1905
— Superfamily Schizochitonoidea Dall, 1889
— Family Schizochitonidae Dall, 1889
— *Incissiochiton* Van Belle, 1985
— *Schizochiton* Gray, 1847
— Suborder Acanthochitonina Bergenhayn, 1930
— Superfamily Mopalioidea Dall, 1889
— Family Tonicellidae Simroth, 1894
— Subfamily Tonicellinae Simroth, 1894
— *Lepidochitona* Gray, 1821
— *Particulazona* Kaas, 1993
— *Boreochiton* Sars, 1878

— *Tonicella* Carpenter, 1873
— *Nuttallina* (Carpenter MS) Dall, 1871
— *Spongioradsia* Pilsbry, 1894
— *Oligochiton* Berry, 1922
— Subfamily Juvenichitoninae Sirenko, 1975
— *Juvenichiton* Sirenko, 1975
— *Micichiton* Sirenko, 1975
— *Nanichiton* Sirenko, 1975
— Family Schizoplacidae Bergenhayn, 1955
— *Schizoplax* Dall, 1878
— Family Mopaliidae Dall, 1889
— Subfamily Heterochitoninae Van Belle, 1978
— *Heterochiton* Fucini, 1912
— *Allochiton* Fucini, 1912
— Subfamily Mopaliinae Dall, 1889
— *Aerilamma* Hull, 1924
— *Guildingia* Pilsbry, 1893
— *Frembleya* H. Adams, 1866
— *Diaphoroplax* Iredale, 1914
— *Plaxiphora* Gray, 1847
— *Placiphorina* Kaas & Van Belle, 1994
— *Nuttallochiton* Plate, 1899
— *Mopalia* Gray, 1847
— *Maorichiton* Iredale, 1914
— *Placiphorella* (Carpenter MS) Dall, 1879
— *Katharina* Gray, 1847
— *Amicula* Gray, 1847
— Superfamily Cryptoplacoidea H. et A. Adams, 1858
— Family Acanthochitonidae Pilsbry, 1893
— Subfamily Acanthochitoninae Pilsbry, 1893
— *Acanthochitona* Gray, 1921
— *Craspedochiton* Shuttleworth, 1853

— *Spongiochiton* (Carpenter MS) Dall, 1882
— *Notoplax* H. Adams, 1861
— *Pseudotonicia* Ashby, 1928
— *Bassethullia* Pilsbry, 1928
— *Americhiton* Watters, 1990
— *Choneplax* (Carpenter MS) Dall, 1882
— *Cryptoconchus* (de Blainville MS) Burrow, 1815
— Subfamily Cryptochitoninae Pilsbry, 1893
— *Cryptochiton* Middendorff, 1847
— Family Hemiarthridae Sirenko, 1997
— *Hemiarthrum* Carpenter in Dall, 1876
— *Weedingia* Kaas, 1988
— Family Choriplacidae Ashby, 1928
— *Choriplax* Pilsbry, 1894
— Family Cryptoplacidae H. et A. Adams, 1858
— *Cryptoplax* de Blainville, 1818

o *Incertae sedis*
— Family Scanochitonidae Bergenhayn, 1955
— *Scanochiton* Bergenhayn, 1955
— Family Olingechitonidae Starobogatov et Sirenko, 1977
— *Olingechiton* Bergenhayn, 1943
— Family Haeggochitonidae Sirenko et Starobogatov, 1977
— *Haeggochiton* Bergenhayn, 1955
— Family Ivoechitonidae Sirenko et Starobogatov, 1977
— *Ivoechiton* Bergenhayn, 1955.

Tusk Shell

The tusk shells or scaphopods are a class of shelled marine molluscs. The scientific name of this class is Scaphopoda, meaning "shovel-footed". Shells of species within this class range from about 0.5 to 15 cm in length. Members of the Order Dentaliida are generally significantly larger than those of the

Order Gadilida. These molluscs live on soft substrates offshore (usually not intertidally). Because of this subtidal habitat and the small size of most species, many beachcombers are unfamiliar with them; their shells are usually not nearly as common or as easily visible in the beach drift as the shells of sea snails and clams. Molecular data suggests that the scaphopods are a sister group to the cephalopods, although higher-level molluscan phylogeny remains somewhat unresolved.

Ecology

Scaphopods feed on microscopic organisms; some supplement their diet of zooplankton with vegetable matter.

Shell Description

The aragonitic shells of scaphopods are conical and curved in a planispiral way, and they are usually whitish in colour. Because of these characteristics, the shell somewhat resembles a miniature elephant's tusk, hence the common name tusk shell. However, unlike an elephant's tusk, the shells of these molluscs are hollow and open at both ends; the opening at the larger end is the main or anterior aperture of the shell. The smaller opening is known as the apical aperture. Some tusk shells are minute, and most are 4 to 6 centimetres (1.6 to 2.4 in) long; however, a few species reach 15 centimetres (5.9 in) in length. The scaphopod shell bears a prominent cross-lamellar layer, and has a bioeroded tip.

Habitat and Distribution

Tusk shells live in seafloor sediment where they feed on detritus, foraminiferans and microscopic animals.

Classification

The group is composed of a two subtaxa, the Dentaliida (which may be paraphyletic) and the monophyletic Gadilida. The differences between the two orders is subtle and hinges on details of the radula and shell.

Anatomy of the Soft Parts

The mantle of a scaphopod is entirely within the shell. The foot extends from the larger end of the shell, and is used to burrow through the substrate. The scaphopod positions itself head down in the substrate, with the apical end of the shell (at the rear of the animal's body) projecting up into the water. Water enters the mantle cavity through the apical aperture, and is wafted along the body surface by cilia. There are no gills; the entire surface of the mantle cavity absorbs oxygen from the water. Unlike most other molluscs, there is no continuous flow of water with a separate exhalant stream. Instead, deoxygenated water is expelled rapidly back through the apical aperture through muscular action once every ten to twelve minutes.

A number of minute tentacles around the foot, called captacula, sift through the sediment and latch onto bits of food, which they then convey to the mouth.

The mouth has a grinding radula that breaks the bit into smaller pieces for digestion. The remainder of the digestive system consists of an oesophagus, stomach, and intestine. A digestive gland secretes enzymes into the stomach, but, unlike some other molluscs, does not digest the food directly itself. The anus opens on the underside of the animal, roughly in the middle of the mantle cavity.

The scaphopod vascular system is rudimentary, lacking both heart and blood vessels; the blood is held in sinuses throughout the body cavity, and is pumped through the body by the rhythmic action of the foot. Metabolic waste is excreted through a pair of nephridia close to the anus.

The nervous system is generally similar to that of gastropods. One pair each of cerebral and pleural ganglia lie close to the oesophagus, and effectively form the animal's brain. A separate set of pedal ganglia lie in the foot, and a pair of visceral ganglia are set further back in the body. Scaphopods have no eyes, or other distinct sensory organs.

Reproduction and Development

Scaphopods have separate sexes, and external fertilisation. They have a single gonad occupying much of the posterior part of the body, and shed their gametes into the water through the nephridium. Once fertilised, the eggs hatch into a free-living trochophore larva, which develops into a veliger larva that more closely resembles the adult, but lacks the extreme elongation of the adult body.

Fossil Record

There is a good fossil record of scaphopods from the Mississippian onwards, making them the youngest molluscan class; but the origin of the group remains contentious. The Ordovician *Rhytiodentalium kentuckyensis* has been interpreted as an early antecedent of the scaphopods, implying an evolutionary succession from ribeirioid rostroconch molluscs such as *Pinnocaris*. However, a competing hypothesis suggests a Devonian/Carboniferous origin from a non-mineralized ancestor, or from a more derived, Devonian, conocardioid rostroconch. As such they were the most recent of all molluscan classes to evolve. They are most closely related to the extinct molluscan class Rostroconchia.

Human Use

The shells of *Dentalium hexagonum*, a scaphopod mollusc, were strung on thread and used by the natives of the Pacific Northwest as shell money. *Dentalium* shells were also used to make belts and headdresses by the Natufian culture of the Middle East, and are a possible indicator of early social stratification. Shells of the species *Dentalium pretiosum* were used as money.

Bivalvia

Bivalvia, commonly called the bivalves, is a taxonomic class of marine and freshwater molluscs that have a laterally compressed body enclosed by a shell in two hinged parts. This class includes the clams, oysters, mussels, scallops and numerous other families. The majority are filter feeders and have no head or rasping tongue. The gills have evolved into ctenidia, specialised organs for feeding and breathing. Most bivalves bury themselves in sediment on the seabed where they are safe from predation. Others lie on the sea floor or attach themselves to rocks or other hard surfaces. A few bore into wood, clay or stone and live inside these substances. Some bivalves, such as the scallops, can swim.

The shell of a bivalve is composed of calcium carbonate and consists of two, usually similar, parts called *valves*. These are joined together at one edge by a flexible ligament that, in conjunction with nearby interlocking "teeth" on the two valves, are known collectively as the hinge. This arrangement allows the shell to be opened and closed without the two halves becoming disarticulated. The shell is typically bilaterally symmetrical, with the hinge lying in the sagittal plane. Adult shell sizes vary from fractions of a millimetre to over a metre in length but the majority of species do not exceed ten centimetres (four inches). Bivalves have long been a part of the diet of coastal communities. Oysters were cultured in ponds by the Romans and mariculture has more recently become an important source of bivalves for food. Modern knowledge of molluscan reproductive cycles has led to the development of hatcheries and new culture techniques.

A better understanding of the hazards of eating raw and undercooked shellfish has led to improved storage and processing. Besides their use as food, oysters are the most common source of natural pearls. The shells of bivalves are used in craftwork and in the manufacture of jewellery and buttons. Bivalves have also been used in the biocontrol of pollution.

Bivalves first appeared in the fossil record in the early Cambrian more than 500 million years ago. The total number of living species is approximately 9,200. These species are placed within 1,260 genera and 106 families. Marine bivalves (including brackish water and estuarine species) represent about 8,000 species, combined in four subclasses and 99 families with 1,100 genera. The largest recent marine families are Veneridae with more than 680 species and the Tellinidae and Lucinidae, each with over 500 species. The freshwater bivalves include seven families, the largest of which is the Unionidae with about 700 species.

Etymology

The taxonomic term Bivalvia was first used by Linnaeus in the 10th edition of his *Systema Naturae* in 1758 to refer to molluscs that had shells composed of two valves. More recently the class was known as Pelecypoda, meaning "axe-foot" (based on the shape of the soft parts of the animal). Other names that have been used for this class include Lamellibranchia (based on the plate-like gill elements, the ctenidium) and Acephala (based on the fact that, unlike other molluscs, these animals have no head). The name *bivalve* is derived from the Latin *bis*, meaning "two", and *valvae*, meaning "leaves of a door". Not all animals that have shells with two hinged parts are classified under Bivalvia; other animals with paired valves include certain gastropods (small sea snails in the family Juliidae), members of the phylum Brachiopoda and the minute crustaceans known as ostracods and conchostrachans.

Mantle and Shell

Near the hinge of the shell is the umbone or beak, a rounded knobbly protuberance. This represents the oldest portion of the shell, extra material later being laid down along the margins on the opposite side. The hinge area is the dorsal region of the shell and the lower margin is the ventral region. The anterior or front of the shell is where the byssus and foot are located and the posterior of the shell is where the siphons are located. When the umbone is uppermost, the valve with the anterior end to the left is considered to be the left valve while the valve with the anterior end to the right is the right valve.

In all molluscs the mantle forms a thin membrane covering the animal's body and extending out from it in flaps or lobes. In bivalves, the mantle lobes secrete the valves, and the mantle crest secretes the whole hinge mechanism consisting of ligament, byssus threads and teeth. Visible on the inside of most empty bivalve valves is a shiny line that runs parallel to the outer margin of the shell and often connects the two adductor muscle scars. This line exists because parallel to the opening edge of the bivalve's shell, the mantle is attached to the shell by a continuous narrow row of minute mantle retractor muscles.

The function of these small muscles is to pull the loose edge of the mantle up out of harm's way when this is necessary because of minor predation attempts. In many bivalves the mantle edges fuse at the posterior end of the shell to form two siphons, through which water is inhaled and expelled for respiration and suspension feeding. There is a pocket-like space into which the siphons fit when they are retracted. This is visible on the inside of the valve as an indentation on the pallial line which is known as the pallial sinus.

The shell is composed of two calcareous valves held together by a ligament. The valves are made of either calcite, as is the case in oysters, or both calcite and aragonite. Sometimes the aragonite forms an inner, nacreous layer, as is the case in the order Pterioida. In other taxa, alternate layers of calcite and aragonite are laid down. The ligament and byssus, if calcified, are composed of aragonite. The outermost layer of the shell is the periostracum, a skin-like layer which is composed of a horny organic substance. The periostracum is secreted in the groove between the outer and middle layers of the mantle, and is usually olive or brown in colour and easily abraded. The outer surface of the valves is often sculpted with clams having fine concentric striations, scallops radial ribs and oysters a latticework of irregular markings.

The shell is added to in two ways; the valves grow larger when more material is secreted by the mantle at the margin of the shell, and the valves themselves thicken gradually throughout the animal's life as more calcareous matter is secreted by the mantle lobes. Although the (sometimes faint) concentric rings on the exterior of a valve are commonly described as "growth rings" or "growth lines", a more accurate method for determining the age of a shell is by cutting a cross section through it and examining the incremental growth bands. Use of this technique has changed views on the longevity of many bivalves.

For example, the soft-shell clam (*Mya arenaria*) was thought to be short-lived, but has now been shown to have a lifespan of at least 28 years. The two valves are held together at a hinge joint by a ligament composed of two keratinised proteins, tensilium and resilium. In different groups of bivalves the ligament can be internal or external in position. The main function of the ligament (as well as joining the valves together) is to passively cause the shell to open.

The shell is actively closed using the adductor muscle or muscles attached to the inner surface of both valves. The position of the muscles is often clearly visible on the inside of empty valves as circular or oval muscle scars.

Along the hinge line of the shell there are often a number of hinge teeth which prevent the valves from moving laterally relative to one another. The arrangement of these teeth is often important in identifying bivalves.

Nervous System

The sedentary habits of the bivalves have led to the development of a nervous system that is less complex than in most other molluscs. The animals have no brain and the nervous system consists of a nerve network and a series of paired ganglia. In all but the most primitive bivalves there are two cerebropleural ganglia on either side of the oesophagus. The cerebral ganglia control the sensory organs while the pleural ganglia supply nerves to the mantle cavity. The pedal ganglia, which control the foot, are at its base, and the visceral ganglia, which can be quite large in swimming bivalves, are under the posterior adductor muscle. These ganglia are both connected to the cerebropleural ganglia by nerve fibres. Bivalves with long siphons may also have siphonal ganglia to control them.

Senses

The sensory organs of bivalves are not well developed and are largely located on the posterior mantle margins. The organs are usually mechanoreceptors or chemoreceptors located in short tentacles.

The chemoreceptor cells taste the water and are sensitive to touch. They are typically found near the siphons, but in some species may fringe the entire mantle cavity. The osphradium is a patch of sensory cells located below the posterior adductor muscle that may serve to taste the water or measure its turbidity, but is probably not homologous with the structure of the same name found in snails and slugs. Statocysts within the organism help the bivalve to sense and correct its orientation. Each statocyst consists of a small sac lined with sensory cilia that detects the movement of a mineral mass, a statolith, under gravity.

In the order Anomalodesmata, the inhalant siphon is surrounded by vibration-sensitive tentacles for detecting prey. Many bivalves have no eyes, but a few members of Arcoidea, Limopsoidea, Mytiloidea, Anomioidea, Ostreoidea and Limoidea have simple eyes on the margin of the mantle. These consist of a pit of photo-sensory cells and a lens. Scallops have more complex eyes with a lens, a two-layered retina and a concave mirror. All bivalves have light-sensitive cells that can detect a shadow falling over the animal.

Muscles

The main muscular system in bivalves is the posterior and anterior adductor muscles, although the anterior muscles may be reduced or even lost in some species. These strong muscles connect the two valves and contract in order to close the shell. They work in opposition to the ligament which tends to pull the valves apart. In sedentary or recumbent bivalves that lie on one valve, such as the oysters and scallops, the anterior adductor muscle has been lost and the posterior muscle is positioned centrally. In file shells that can swim by flapping their valves, there is also a single, central adductor muscle. These muscles are composed of two types of muscle fibre, striated muscle bundles for fast actions and smooth muscle bundles for maintaining a steady pull. The mantle suspender muscles attach the mantle to the shell and leave an arc-shaped scar on the inside of the valve, the pallial line. The paired pedal protractor and retractor muscles operate the animal's foot. Some bivalves, such as oysters and most scallops, are unable to extend their foot and in them, these muscles are absent. Other paired muscles control the siphons and the byssus.

Circulation and Respiration

Bivalves have an open circulatory system that bathes the organs in hemolymph. The heart has three chambers: two auricles receiving blood from the gills, and a single ventricle. The ventricle is muscular and pumps hemolymph into the aorta, and then to the rest of the body. Some bivalves have a single aorta, but most also have a second, usually smaller, aorta serving the hind parts of the animal.

Oxygen is absorbed into the hemolymph in the gills, which have a large surface area and hang down into the mantle cavity. This provides a secondary respiratory surface and is well supplied with capillaries.

In species with no gills, such as the subclass Anomalodesmata, the wall of the mantle cavity is the only organ involved in respiration. Bivalves adapted to tidal environments can survive for several hours out of water by closing their shells tightly. Some freshwater species, when exposed to the air, can gape the shell slightly and gas exchange can take place.

The hemolymph usually lacks any respiratory pigment, although members of the families Arcidae and Limidae are known to possess haemoglobin dissolved directly into the serum. In the carnivorous genus *Poromya*, the hemolymph has red amoebocytes containing a haemoglobin pigment.

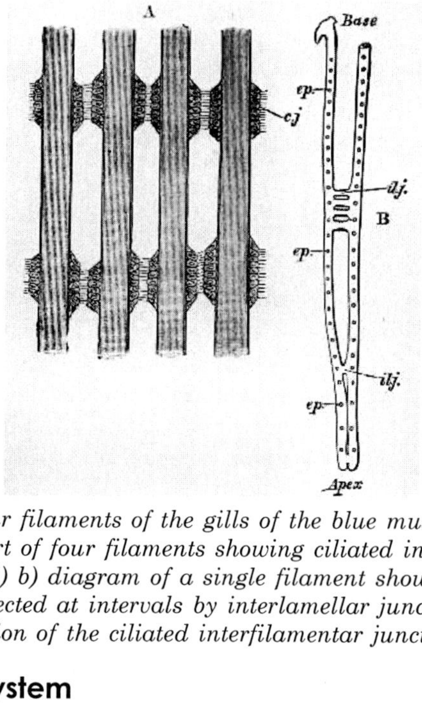

Figure: *Four filaments of the gills of the blue mussel (Mytilus edulis) a) part of four filaments showing ciliated interfilamentar junctions (cj) b) diagram of a single filament showing the two lamellae connected at intervals by interlamellar junctions (ilj) and the position of the ciliated interfilamentar junctions (cp)*

Digestive System

Modes of Feeding

Most bivalves are filter feeders, using their gills to capture particulate food such as phytoplankton from the water. The Protobranchs feed in a different way, scraping detritus from the seabed, and this may be the original mode of feeding used by all bivalves before the gills became adapted for filter feeding. These primitive bivalves hold onto the substratum with a pair of tentacles at the edge of the mouth, each of which has a single palp, or flap. The tentacles are covered in mucus, which traps the food, and cilia, which transport the particles back to the palps. These then sort the particles, rejecting those that are unsuitable or too large to digest, and conveying others to the mouth. In the Filibranchia and Eulamellibranchia, water is drawn into the shell from the posterior ventral surface of the animal, passes upwards through the gills and doubles back to be expelled just above the intake. In burrowing species, there may be two elongated, retractable siphons reaching up to the seabed, one each for the inhalant and exhalant streams of water. The gills of filter-feeding bivalves are known as ctenidia and have become highly modified to increase their ability to capture food. For example, the cilia on the gills, which originally served to remove unwanted sediment, have become adapted to capture food particles, and transport them in a steady stream of mucus to the mouth. The filaments of the gills are also much longer than those in more primitive bivalves, and are folded over to create a groove through which food can be transported. The structure of the gills varies considerably, and can serve as a useful means for classifying bivalves into groups.

A few bivalves, such as the granular poromya (*Poromya granulata*), are carnivorous, eating much larger prey than the tiny microalgae consumed by other bivalves. In these animals, the gills are relatively small, and form a perforated barrier separating the main mantle cavity from a smaller chamber through which the water is exhaled. Muscles draw water in through the inhalant siphon which is modified into a cowl-shaped organ, sucking in small crustaceans and worms at the same time.

The siphon can be retracted quickly and inverted, bringing the prey within reach of the mouth. The gut is modified so that large food particles can be digested. The unusual genus, *Entovalva*, is endosymbiontic, being found only in the oesophagus of sea cucumbers. It has mantle folds that completely surround its small valves. When the sea cucumber sucks in sediment, the bivalve allows the water to pass over its gills and extracts fine organic particles. To prevent itself from being swept away, it attaches itself with byssal threads to the host's throat. The sea cucumber is unharmed.

Digestive Tract

The digestive tract of typical bivalves consists of an oesophagus, stomach, and intestine. A number of digestive glands open into the stomach, often via a pair of diverticula;

these secrete enzymes to digest food in the stomach, but also include cells that phagocytose food particles, and digest them intracellularly. In filter-feeding bivalves, an elongated rod of solidified mucus referred to as the "crystalline style" projects into the stomach from an associated sac. Cilia in the sac cause the style to rotate, winding in a stream of food-containing mucus from the mouth, and churning the stomach contents.

This constant motion propels food particles into a sorting region at the rear of the stomach, which distributes smaller particles into the digestive glands, and heavier particles into the intestine. Waste material is consolidated in the rectum and voided as pellets into the exhalent water stream through an anal pore.

Feeding and digestion are synchronized with diurnal and tidal cycles. Carnivorous bivalves have a greatly reduced style, and a chitinous gizzard that helps grind up the food before digestion. In other ways their gut is similar to that of filter-feeding bivalves.

Excretory System

Like most other molluscs, the excretory organs of bivalves are a pair of nephridia. Each of these consists of a long, looped, glandular tube, which opens into the body cavity just beneath the heart, and a bladder to store urine. There are also pericardial glands, either lining the auricles of the heart or attached to the pericardium, which serve as extra filtration organs. Metabolic waste is voided from the bladders through a pair of openings near the front of the upper part of the mantle cavity, from where it joins the stream of exhalant water.

Reproduction and Development

The sexes are usually separate in bivalves but some hermaphroditism is known. The gonads are located close to the intestines, and either open into the nephridia, or through a separate pore into the mantle cavity.

The ripe gonads of male and females release sperm and eggs into the water column. Spawning may take place continually or be triggered by environmental factors such as day length, water temperature or the presence of sperm in the water. Some species are "dribble spawners" but others release their gametes in batches or all at once. Mass spawning events sometimes take place when all the bivalves in an area synchronise their release of spawn. Fertilization is usually external. Typically, there is a short stage lasting a few hours or days before the eggs hatch into trochophore larvae. These later develop into veliger larvae which settle on the seabed and undergo metamorphosis into juveniles known as spat. In some species, such as those in the genus *Lasaea*, females draw water containing sperm in through their inhalant siphons and fertilisation is inside the female. These species then brood the young inside their mantle cavity, eventually releasing them into the water column as veliger larvae or as crawl-away juveniles.

Most of the bivalve larvae that hatch from eggs in the water column feed on diatoms or other phytoplankton. In temperate regions, about 25% of species are lecithotrophic, depending on nutrients stored in the yolk of the egg where the main energy source is lipids. The longer the period is before the larva first feeds, the larger the egg and yolk need to be. The reproductive cost of producing these energy-rich eggs is high and they are usually smaller in number. For example, the Baltic tellin (*Macoma balthica*) produces few, high-energy eggs. The larvae hatching out of these rely on the energy reserves and do not feed. After about four days they become D-stage larvae, the stage at which they first develop hinged, D-shaped valves. These larvae have a relatively small dispersal potential before settling out. The common mussel (*Mytilus edulis*) produces ten times as many eggs that hatch into larvae and soon need to feed in order to survive and grow. They can disperse more widely as they remain planktonic for a much longer time.

Freshwater bivalves in the order Unionoida have a different life cycle. Sperm is drawn into a female's gills with the inhalant water and internal fertilization takes place. The eggs hatch into glochidia larvae that develop within the female's shell. Later they are released and attach themselves parasitically to the gills or fins of a fish host. After several weeks they drop off their host, undergo metamorphosis and develop into juveniles on the substrate. An advantage of this to the molluscs is that they may be able to disperse upstream with their temporary hosts rather than being constantly swept downstream by the water flow. Some of the species in the freshwater mussel family, Unionidae, commonly known as *pocketbook mussels*, have evolved an unusual reproductive strategy. The female's mantle protrudes from the shell and develops into an imitation small fish, complete with fish-like markings and false eyes. This decoy moves in the current and attracts the attention of real fish. Some fish see the decoy as prey, while others see a conspecific. Whatever they see, they approach for a closer look and the mussel releases huge numbers of larvae from its gills, dousing the inquisitive fish with its tiny, parasitic young. These glochidia larvae are drawn into the fish's gills where they attach and trigger a tissue response that forms a small cyst around each larva. The larvae then feed by breaking down and digesting the tissue of the fish within the cysts. After a few weeks they release themselves from the cysts and fall to the stream bed as juvenile molluscs. The fish are relatively unharmed.

Comparison with Brachiopods

Brachiopods are shelled marine organisms that superficially resembled bivalves in that they were of similar size and had a hinged shell in two parts. However, brachiopods evolved from a very different ancestral line, and the resemblance to bivalves only arose because of a similar lifestyle.

The differences between the two groups are due to their separate ancestral origins. Different initial structures have been adapted to solve the same problems, a case of convergent evolution. In modern times, brachiopods are not as common as bivalves.

Both groups have a shell consisting of two valves, but the organisation of the shell is quite different in the two groups. In brachiopods, the two valves are positioned on the dorsal and ventral surfaces of the body, while in bivalves, the valves are on the left and right sides of the body, and are normally mirror images of one other.

Brachiopods have a lophophore, a coiled, rigid cartilaginous internal apparatus adapted for filter feeding, a feature shared with two other major groups of marine invertebrates, the bryozoans and the phoronids. Brachiopod shells are often made of calcium phosphate as well as calcium carbonate, whereas bivalve shells are composed entirely of calcium carbonate.

Evolutionary History

The Cambrian explosion took place 543 to 525 million years ago. In this geologically brief period all the major animal phyla appeared and these included the first creatures with mineralized skeletons. Brachiopods and bivalves made their appearance at this time and left their fossilized remains behind in the rocks. The fossils of both were formed when the sediment in which they were buried hardened into rock. Often it is the impression made by the valves that remains as a fossil rather than the valves themselves.

During the Early Ordovician there was a great increase in the diversity of bivalve species and the dysodont, heterodont and taxodont dentitions evolved. By the early Silurian, the gills were becoming adapted for filter feeding and during the Devonian and Carboniferous periods siphons first appeared which, with the newly developed muscular foot, allowed the animals to bury themselves deep in the sediment.

By the middle of the Paleozoic, around 400 million years ago, the brachiopods were among the most abundant filter feeders in the ocean and over 12,000 fossil species are recognised. By the Permian-Triassic extinction event 250 million years ago, bivalves were undergoing a huge radiation of diversity. The bivalves were hard hit by this event but re-established themselves and thrived during the Triassic period that followed. In contrast, the brachiopods lost 95% of their species diversity. Scientists have speculated that the ability of some bivalves to burrow and thus avoid predators was a major factor in their success. Other new adaptations within various families allowed species to occupy previously unused evolutionary niches. These included increasing relative buoyancy in soft sediments by developing spines on the shell, gaining the ability to swim, and in a few cases, adopting predatory habits.

It was for a long time thought that bivalves were better adapted to aquatic life than brachiopods were, out-competing and relegating them to minor niches in later ages. These two taxa appeared in textbooks as an example of replacement by competition.

Evidence given for this included the fact that bivalves needed less food to subsist because of their energetically efficient ligament-muscle system for opening and closing valves. An alternative view is that the prominence of modern bivalves over brachiopods might merely be due to chance disparities in their response to extinction events.

Distribution

The bivalves are a highly successful class of invertebrates found in aquatic habitats throughout the world. Most are infaunal and live buried in sediment on the seabed, or in the sediment in freshwater habitats. A large number of bivalve species are found in the intertidal and sublittoral zones of the oceans. A sandy sea beach may superficially appear to be devoid of life, but there is often a very large number of bivalves and other invertebrates living beneath the surface of the sand. On a large beach in South Wales, careful sampling produced an estimate of 1.44 million cockles (*Cerastoderma edule*) per acre of beach. Bivalves inhabit the tropics as well as temperate and boreal waters. A number of species can survive and even flourish in extreme conditions.

They are abundant in the Arctic, about 140 species being known from that zone. The Antarctic scallop, *Adamussium colbecki*, lives under the sea ice at the other end of the globe, where the sub-zero temperatures mean that growth rates are very slow. The giant mussel, *Bathymodiolus thermophilus*, and the giant white clam, *Calyptogena magnifica*, both live clustered around hydrothermal vents at abyssal depths in the Pacific Ocean. They have chemosymbiotic bacteria in their gills that oxidise hydrogen sulphide, and the molluscs absorb nutrients synthesized by these bacteria. The saddle oyster, *Enigmonia aenigmatica*, is a marine species that could be considered amphibious. It lives above the high tide mark in the tropical Indo-Pacific on the underside of mangrove leaves, on mangrove branches and on sea walls in the splash zone. Some freshwater bivalves have very restricted ranges. For example, the Ouachita creekshell mussel, *Villosa arkansasensis*, is known only from the streams of the Ouachita Mountains in Arkansas and Oklahoma, and like several other freshwater mussel species from the southeastern USA, it is in danger of extinction.

In contrast, a few species of freshwater bivalves, including the golden mussel (*Limnoperna fortunei*), are dramatically increasing their ranges. The golden mussel has spread from south-east Asia to Argentina, where it has become an invasive species. Another well-travelled freshwater bivalve, the zebra mussel (*Dreissena polymorpha*) originated in southeastern Russia, and has been accidentally introduced to inland waterways in North America and Europe, where the species damages water installations and disrupts local ecosystems.

Behaviour

Most bivalves adopt a sedentary or even sessile life style, often spending their whole lives in the area in which they first settled as juveniles. The majority of bivalves are infaunal, living under the seabed, buried in soft substrates such as sand, silt, mud, gravel or coral fragments. Many of these live in the intertidal zone where the sediment remains damp even when the tide is out. When buried in the sediment, burrowing bivalves are protected from the pounding of waves, desiccation and overheating during low tide, and variations in salinity caused by rainwater. They are also out of the reach of many predators. Their general strategy is to extend their siphons to the surface for feeding and respiration during high tide, but to descend to greater depths or keep their shell tightly shut when the tide goes out. They use their muscular foot to dig into the substrate.

To do this, the animal relaxes its adductor muscles and opens its shell wide to anchor itself in position while it extends its foot downwards into the substrate. Then it dilates the tip of its foot, retracts the adductor muscles to close the shell, shortens its foot and draws itself downwards. This series of actions is repeated to dig deeper. Other bivalves, such as mussels, attach themselves to hard surfaces using tough byssus threads made of keratin and proteins.

They are more exposed to attack by predators than the burrowing bivalves. Certain carnivorous gastropod snails such as whelks (Buccinidae) and murex snails (Muricidae) feed on bivalves by boring into their shells. The dog whelk (*Nucella lamellosa*) drills a hole with its radula assisted by a shell-dissolving secretion. The dog whelk then inserts its extendible proboscis and sucks out the body contents of the victim, which is typically a blue mussel. The whelk needs a few hours to penetrate the shell and thus living in the littoral zone is an advantage to the bivalve because the gastropod can attempt to bore through the shell only when the tide is in.

Some bivalves, including the true oysters, the jewel boxes, the jingle shells, the thorny oysters and the kitten's paws, cement themselves to stones, rock or larger dead shells. In oysters the lower valve may be almost flat while the upper valve develops layer upon layer of thin horny material reinforced with calcium carbonate. Oysters sometimes occur in dense beds in the neritic zone and, like most bivalves, are filter feeders. Although many non-sessile bivalves use their muscular foot to move around, or to dig, members of the freshwater family Sphaeriidae are exceptional in that these small clams climb about quite nimbly on weeds using their long and flexible foot. The European fingernail clam (*Sphaerium corneum*), for example, climbs around on water weeds at the edges of lakes and ponds; this enables the clam to find the best position for filter feeding.

Predators and Defence

The thick shell and rounded shape of bivalves make them awkward for potential predators to tackle. Nevertheless, a number of different creatures include them in their diet. Many species of demersal fish feed on them including the common carp (*Cyprinus carpio*), which is being used in the upper Mississippi River to try to control the invasive zebra mussel (*Dreissena polymorpha*). Birds such as the Eurasian Oystercatcher (*Haematopus ostralegus*) have specially adapted beaks which can pry open their shells. The herring gull (*Larus argentatus*) sometimes drops heavy shells onto rocks in order to crack them open. Sea otters feed on a variety of bivalve species and have been observed to use stones balanced on their chests as anvils on which to crack open the shells. The Pacific walrus (*Odobenus rosmarus divergens*) is one of the main predators feeding on bivalves in Arctic waters. Shellfish have formed part of the human diet since prehistoric times, a fact evidenced by the remains of mollusc shells found in ancient middens. Examinations of these deposits in Peru has provided a means of dating long past El Niño events because of the disruption these caused to bivalve shell growth.

Invertebrate predators include crabs, starfish and octopuses. Crabs crack the shells with their pincers and starfish use their water vascular system to force the valves apart and then insert part of their stomach between the valves to digest the bivalve's body. It has been found experimentally that both crabs and starfish preferred molluscs that are attached by byssus threads to ones that are cemented to the substrate. This was probably because they could manipulate the shells and open them more easily when they could tackle them from different angles. Octopuses either pull bivalves apart by force, or they bore a hole into the shell and insert a digestive fluid before sucking out the liquified contents. Razor shells can dig themselves into the sand with great speed to escape predation. When a Pacific razor clam (*Siliqua patula*) is laid on the surface of the beach it can bury itself completely in seven seconds and the Atlantic jackknife clam, *Ensis directus*, can do the same within fifteen seconds.

Scallops and file clams can swim by opening and closing their valves rapidly; water is ejected on either side of the hinge area and they move with the flapping valves in front. Scallops have simple eyes around the margin of the mantle and can clap their valves shut to move sharply, hinge first, to escape from danger. Cockles can use their foot to move across the seabed or leap away from threats. The foot is first extended before being contracted suddenly when it acts like a spring, projecting the animal forwards. In many bivalves that have siphons, they can be retracted back into the safety of the shell. If the siphons inadvertently get attacked by a predator, they snap off. The animal can regenerate them later, a process that starts when the cells close to the damaged site become activated and remodel the tissue back to its pre-existing form and size.

File shells such as *Limaria fragilis* can produce a noxious secretion when stressed. It has numerous tentacles which fringe its mantle and protrude some distance from the shell when it is feeding. If attacked, it sheds tentacles in a process known as autotomy. The toxin released by this is distasteful and the detached tentacles continue to writhe which may also serve to distract potential predators.

Mariculture

European flat oysters (*Ostrea edulis*) were first farmed by the Romans in shallow ponds and similar techniques are still in use. Seed oysters are either raised in a hatchery or harvested from the wild. Hatchery production provides some control of the broodstock but remains problematic because disease-resistant strains of this oyster have not yet been developed. Wild spats are harvested either by broadcasting empty mussel shells on the seabed or by the use of long, small-mesh nets filled with mussel shells supported on steel frames. The oyster larvae preferentially settle out on the mussel shells. Juvenile oysters are then grown on in nursery trays and are transferred to open waters when they reach 5 to 6 millimetres (0.20 to 0.24 in) in length. Many juveniles are further reared off the seabed in suspended rafts, on floating trays or cemented to ropes. Here they are largely free from bottom-dwelling predators such as starfish and crabs but more labour is required to tend them. They can be harvested by hand when they reach a suitable size. Other juveniles are laid directly on the seabed at the rate of 50 to 100 kilograms (110 to 220 lb) per hectare. They grow on for about two years before being harvested by dredging. Survival rates are low at about 5%.

The Pacific oyster (*Crassostrea gigas*) is cultivated by similar methods but in larger volumes and in many more regions of the world. This oyster originated in Japan where it has been cultivated for many centuries. It is an estuarine species and prefers salinities of 20 to 25 parts per thousand. Breeding programmes have produced improved stock that is available from hatcheries. A single female oyster can produce 50–80 million eggs in a batch so the selection of broodstock is of great importance. The larvae are grown on in tanks of static or moving water. They are fed high quality microalgae and diatoms and grow fast. At metamorphosis the juveniles may be allowed to settle on PVC sheets or pipes, or crushed shell.

In some cases, they continue their development in "upwelling culture" in large tanks of moving water rather than being allowed to settle on the bottom. They then may be transferred to transitional, nursery beds before being moved to their final rearing quarters. Culture there takes place on the bottom, in plastic trays, in mesh bags, on rafts or on long lines, either in shallow water or in the intertidal zone. The oysters are ready for harvesting in 18 to 30 months depending on the size required. Similar techniques are used in different parts of the world to cultivate other species including the Sydney rock oyster (*Saccostrea commercialis*), the Northern quahog (*Mercenaria mercenaria*), the blue mussel (*Mytilus edulis*), the Mediterranean mussel (*Mytilus galloprovincialis*), the New Zealand green-lipped mussel (*Perna canaliculus*), the grooved carpet shell (*Ruditapes decussatus*), the Japanese carpet shell (*Venerupis philippinarum*), the pullet carpet shell (*Venerupis pullastra*) and the Yesso scallop (*Patinopecten yessoensis*).

Production of bivalve molluscs by mariculture in 2010 was 12,913,199 tons, up from 8,320,724 tons in 2000. Culture of clams, cockles and ark shells more than doubled over this time period from 2,354,730 to 4,885,179 tons. Culture of mussels over the same period grew from 1,307,243 to 1,812,371 tons, of oysters from 3,610,867 to 4,488,544 tons and of scallops from 1,047,884 to 1,727,105 tons.

Use as Food

Bivalves have been an important source of food for humans at least since Roman times and empty shells found in middens at archaeological sites are evidence of earlier consumption. Oysters, scallops, clams, ark clams, mussels and cockles are the most commonly consumed kinds of bivalve, and are eaten cooked or raw.

In 1950, the year in which the Food and Agriculture Organisation (FAO) started making such information available, world trade in bivalve molluscs was 1,007,419 tons. By 2010, world trade in bivalves had risen to 14,616,172 tons, up from 10,293,607 tons a decade earlier. The figures included 5,554,348 (3,152,826) tons of clams, cockles and ark shells, 1,901,314 (1,568,417) tons of mussels, 4,592,529 (3,858,911) tons of oysters and 2,567,981 (1,713,453) tons of scallops. China increased its consumption 400-fold during the period 1970 to 1997.

It has been known for more than a century that consumption of raw or insufficiently cooked shellfish can be associated with infectious diseases. These are caused either by bacteria naturally present in the sea such as *Vibrio spp.* or by viruses and bacteria from sewage effluent that sometimes contaminates coastal waters. As filter feeders, bivalves pass large quantities of water through their gills, filtering out the organic particles, including the microbial pathogens. These are retained in the animals' tissues and become concentrated in their liver-like digestive glands. Another possible source of contamination occurs when bivalves contain marine biotoxins as a result of ingesting numerous dinoflagellates. These microalgae are not associated with sewage but occur unpredictably as algal blooms. Large areas of a sea or lake may change colour as a result of the proliferation of millions of single-cell algae, and this condition is known as a red tide.

Viral and Bacterial Infections

In 1816 in France, a physician, J. P. A. Pasquier, described an outbreak of typhoid linked to the consumption of raw oysters. The first report of this kind in the United states was in Connecticut in 1894. As sewage treatment programmes became more prevalent in the late 19th century, more outbreaks took place. This may have been because sewage was released through outlets into the sea providing more food for bivalves in estuaries and coastal habitats. A causal link between the bivalves and the illness was not easy to demonstrate because the illness might come on days or even weeks after the ingestion of the contaminated shellfish. One viral pathogen is the *Norwalk* virus. This is resistant to treatment with chlorine-containing chemicals and may be present in the marine environment even when coliform bacteria have been killed by the treatment of sewage.

In 1975 in the United States, a serious outbreak of oyster-vectored disease was caused by *Vibrio vulnificus*. Although the number of victims was low, the mortality rate was high at 50%. About 10 cases have occurred annually since then and further research needs to be done to establish the epidemiology of the infections. The cases peak in mid-summer and autumn with no cases being reported in mid winter so there may be a link between the temperature at which the oysters are held between harvesting and consumption. In 1978, an oyster-associated gastrointestinal infection affecting more than 2,000 people occurred in Australia.

The causative agent was found to be the Norwalk virus and the epidemic caused major economic difficulties to the oyster farming industry in the country. In 1988, an outbreak of Hepatitis A associated with the consumption of clams

(*Anadara subcrenata*) took place in the Shanghai area of China. An estimated 290,000 people were infected and there were 47 deaths. In the United States and the European Union, since the early 1990s regulations have been in place that are designed to prevent shellfish from contaminated waters entering the food chain. This has meant that there is sometimes a shortage of regulated shellfish, with consequent higher prices. This has led to illegal harvesting and sale of shellfish on the black market, which can be a health hazard.

Paralytic Shellfish Poisoning

Paralytic shellfish poisoning (PSP) is primarily caused by the consumption of bivalves that have accumulated toxins by feeding on toxic dinoflagellates, single-celled protists found naturally in the sea and inland waters. Saxitoxin is the most virulent of these. In mild cases, PSP causes tingling, numbness, sickness and diarrhoea. In more severe cases, the muscles of the chest wall may be affected leading to paralysis and even death. In 1937, researchers in California established the connection between blooms of these phytoplankton and PSP. The biotoxin remains potent even when the shellfish are well-cooked. In the United States, there is a regulatory limit of 80 μg/g of saxitoxin equivalent in shellfish meat.

Amnesic Shellfish Poisoning

Amnesic shellfish poisoning (ASP) was first reported in eastern Canada in 1987. It is caused by the substance domoic acid found in certain diatoms of the genus *Pseudo-nitzschia*. Bivalves can become toxic when they filter these microalgae out of the water. Domoic acid is a low-molecular weight amino acid that is able to destroy brain cells causing memory loss, gastroenteritis, long-term neurological problems or death. In an outbreak in western USA in 1993, finfish were also implicated as vectors, and sea birds and mammals suffered neurological symptoms. In the United States and Canada, a regulatory limit of 20 μg/g of domoic acid in shellfish meat is set.

Use in Controlling Pollution

When they live in polluted waters, bivalve molluscs have a tendency to accumulate substances such as heavy metals and persistent organic pollutants in their tissues. This is because they ingest the chemicals as they feed but their enzyme systems are not capable of metabolising them and as a result, the levels build up. This may be a health hazard for the molluscs themselves and for humans who eat them. It also has certain advantages in that bivalves can be used in monitoring the presence and quantity of pollutants in their environment. There are limitations to the use of bivalves as bioindicators. The level of pollutants found in the tissues varies with species, age, size, time of year and other factors. The quantities of pollutants in the water may vary and the molluscs may reflect past rather than present values. In a study of several bivalve species present in lagoons in Ghana it was found that the findings could be anomalous.

Levels of zinc and iron tended to rise in the wet season due to run-off from the galvanized roofing sheets used in many of the houses. Cadmium levels were lower in young animals than in older ones because they were growing so fast that, despite the fact that their bodies were accumulating the metal, the concentration in their tissues reduced. In a study near Vladivostok it was found that the level of pollutants in the bivalve tissues did not always reflect the high levels in the surrounding sediment in such places as harbours. The reason for this was thought to be that the bivalves in these locations did not need to filter so much water as elsewhere because of the water's high nutritional content. A study of nine different bivalves with widespread distributions in tropical marine waters concluded that the mussel, *Trichomya hirsuta*, most nearly reflected in its tissues the level of heavy metals (Pb, Cd, Cu, Zn, Co, Ni, and Ag) in its environment. In this species there was a linear relationship between the sedimentary levels and the tissue concentration of all the metals except zinc. In the Persian Gulf, the Atlantic pearl-oyster (*Pinctada radiata*) is considered to be a useful bioindicator of heavy metals.

Crushed shells, available as a by-product of the seafood canning industry, can be used to remove pollutants from water. It has been found that, as long as the water is maintained at an alkaline pH, crushed shells will remove cadmium, lead and other heavy metals from contaminated waters by swapping the calcium in their constituent aragonite for the heavy metal, and retaining these pollutants in a solid form. The rock oyster

(*Saccostrea cucullata*) has been shown to reduce the levels of copper and cadmium in contaminated waters in the Persian Gulf. The live animals acted as biofilters, selectively removing these metals, and the dead shells also had the ability to reduce their concentration.

Other Uses

Conchology is the scientific study of mollusc shells, but the term conchologist is also sometimes used to describe a collector of shells. Many people pick up shells on the beach or purchase them and display them in their homes. There are many private and public collections of mollusc shells, but the largest one in the world is at the Smithsonian Institution, which houses in excess of 20 million specimens. Shells are used decoratively in many ways. They can be pressed into concrete or plaster to make decorative paths, steps or walls and can be used to embellish picture frames, mirrors or other craft items. They can be stacked up and glued together to make ornaments.

They can be pierced and threaded onto necklaces or made into other forms of jewellery. Shells have had various uses in the past as body decorations, utensils, scrapers and cutting implements. Carefully cut and shaped shell tools dating back 32,000 years have been found in a cave in Indonesia. In this region, shell technology may have been developed in preference to the use of stone or bone implements, perhaps because of the scarcity of suitable rock materials.

The indigenous peoples of the Americas living near the east coast used pieces of shell as wampum. The channeled whelk (*Busycotypus canaliculatus*) and the quahog (*Mercenaria mercenaria*) were used to make white and purple traditional patterns. The shells were cut, rolled, polished and drilled before being strung together and woven into belts. These were used for personal, social and ceremonial purposes and also, at a later date, for currency.

The Winnebago Tribe from Wisconsin had numerous uses for freshwater mussels including using them as spoons, cups, ladles and utensils. They notched them to provide knives, graters and saws. They carved them into fish hooks and lures. They incorporated powdered shell into clay to temper their pottery vessels. They used them as scrapers for removing flesh from hides and for separating the scalps of their victims. They used shells as scoops for gouging out fired logs when building canoes and they drilled holes in them and fitted wooden handles for tilling the ground. Buttons have traditionally been made from seashells. At first they were used decoratively rather than as fasteners and the earliest known example dates back five thousand years and was found at Mohenjo-daro in the Indus Valley.

Sea silk is a fine fabric woven from the byssus threads of bivalves, particularly the pen shell (*Pinna nobilis*). It used to be produced in the Mediterranean region where these shells are endemic. It was an expensive fabric and overfishing has much reduced populations of the pen shell. There is mention in the Greek text on the Rosetta Stone (196 BCE) of this cloth being used to pay taxes. Crushed shells are added as a calcareous supplement to the diet of laying poultry. Oyster shell and cockle shell are often used for this purpose and are obtained as a by-product from other industries.

Pearls and Mother-of-Pearl

Mother-of-pearl or nacre is the naturally occurring lustrous layer that lines some mollusc shells. It is used to make pearl buttons and in artisan craftwork to make organic jewellery. It has traditionally been inlaid into furniture and boxes, particularly in China. It has been used to decorate musical instruments, watches, pistols, fans and other products. The import and export of goods made with nacre are controlled in many countries under the International Convention of Trade in Endangered Species of Wild Fauna and Flora.

A pearl is created in the mantle of a mollusc when an irritant particle is surrounded by layers of nacre. Although most bivalves can create pearls, oysters in the family Pteriidae and freshwater mussels in the family Unionidae and Margaritiferidae are the main source of commercially available pearls because the calcareous concretions produced by most other species have no lustre.

Finding pearls inside oysters is a very chancy business as hundreds of shells may need to be prised open before a single pearl can be found. Most pearls are now obtained from cultured shells where an irritant substance has been purposefully introduced to induce the formation of a pearl. A "mabe" (irregular) pearl can be grown by the insertion of an implant, usually made of plastic, under a flap of the mantle and next to the mother-of-pearl interior of the shell. A more difficult procedure is the grafting of a piece of oyster mantle into the gonad of an adult specimen together with the insertion of a shell bead nucleus. This produces a superior, spherical pearl. The animal can be opened to extract the pearl after about two years and reseeded so that it produces another pearl. Pearl oyster farming and pearl culture is an important industry in Japan and many other countries bordering the Indian and Pacific Oceans.

Symbolism

The scallop is the symbol of St James and is called "La coquille Saint-Jacques" in French. It is an emblem carried by pilgrims on their way to the shrine of Santiago de Compostela in Galicia. The shell became associated with the pilgrimage and came to be used as a symbol showing hostelries along the route and later as a sign of hospitality, food and lodging elsewhere. Roman myth has it that Venus, the goddess of love, was born in the sea and emerged accompanied by fish and dolphins, with Botticelli depicting her as arriving in a scallop shell. The Romans revered her and erected shrines in her honour in their gardens, praying to her to provide water and verdant growth. From this, the scallop and other bivalve shells came to be used as a symbol for fertility. Its depiction is used in architecture, furniture and fabric design and it is the logo of Royal Dutch Shell, the global oil and gas company.

Historical Taxonomy

Many systems have been developed for the classification of bivalves but for the past two centuries, no consensus has existed on bivalve phylogeny. In the earlier taxonomic systems, experts used only one characteristic feature for their taxonomic system, choosing between shell morphology, hinge type or gill type. Conflicting naming schemes proliferated due to taxonomies based on single organ systems. One of the most widely accepted systems was that put forward by Norman D. Newell in Part N of the *Treatise on Invertebrate Paleontology*, which employed a classification system based on general shell shape, microstructures and hinge configuration. Because features such as hinge morphology, dentition, mineralogy, shell morphology and shell composition change slowly over time, these characteristics can be used to define major taxonomic groups. There are numerous fossil lineages, however DNA sequence data is only of limited use in classifying extinct species because the DNA available from fossil specimens is often of low quality, and may have been contaminated.

Since the year 2000, taxonomic studies using cladistical analyses of multiple organ systems, shell morphology (including fossil species) and modern molecular phylogenetics have resulted in the drawing up of what experts believe is a more accurate phylogeny of the Bivalvia. Based upon these studies, a new proposed classification system for the Bivalvia was published in 2010 by Bieler, Carter & Coan. In 2012, this new system was adopted by the World Register of Marine Species (WoRMS) for the classification of the Bivalvia. Some experts still maintain that Anomalodesmacea should be considered a separate subclass, whereas the new system treats it as the order Anomalodesmata, within the Heterodonta. Molecular phylogeny work continues, further clarifying which organisms are most closely related and thus refining the taxonomy of the Bivalvia.1935 taxonomy

In his 1935 work *Handbuch der systematischen Weichtierkunde* (Handbook of Systematic Malacology), Johannes Thiele introduced a mollusc taxonomy based upon the 1909 work by Cossmann and Peyrot. Thiele's system divided the bivalves into three orders. *Taxodonta* consisted of forms that had taxodont dentition, with a series of small parallel teeth perpendicular to the hinge line. *Anisomyaria* consisted of forms that had either a single adductor muscle or one adductor muscle much smaller than the other. *Eulamellibranchiata* consisted of forms with ctenidial gills. The Eulamellibranchiata was further divided into four suborders: *Schizodonta*, *Heterodonta*, *Adapedonta* and *Anomalodesmata.*

Taxonomy Based upon Gill Morphology

An alternative systematic scheme exists using gill morphology. This distinguishes between Protobranchia, Filibranchia and Eulamellibranchia. The first corresponds to Newell's Palaeotaxodonta and Cryptodonta, the second to his

Pteriomorphia, with the last corresponding to all other groups. In addition, Franc separated the Septibranchia from his eulamellibranchs because of the morphological differences between them. The septibranchs belong to the superfamily Poromyoidea and are carnivorous, having a muscular septum instead of filamentous gills.

Gastropoda

The Gastropoda or gastropods, more commonly known as snails and slugs, are a large taxonomic class within the phylum Mollusca. The class Gastropoda includes snails and slugs of all kinds and all sizes from microscopic to quite large. There are huge numbers of sea snails and sea slugs, as well as freshwater snails and freshwater limpets, and land snails and land slugs. The class Gastropoda contains a vast total of named species, second only to the insects in overall number. The fossil history of this class goes back to the Late Cambrian. There are 611 families of gastropods, of which 202 families are extinct, being found only in the fossil record. Gastropoda (previously known as univalves and sometimes spelled Gasteropoda) are a major part of the phylum Mollusca and are the most highly diversified class in the phylum, with 60,000 to 80,000 living snail and slug species. The anatomy, behaviour, feeding and reproductive adaptations of gastropods vary significantly from one clade or group to another. Therefore, it is difficult to state many generalities for all gastropods.

The class Gastropoda has an extraordinary diversification of habitats. Representatives live in gardens, in woodland, in deserts, and on mountains; in small ditches, great rivers and lakes; in estuaries, mudflats, the rocky intertidal, the sandy subtidal, in the abyssal depths of the oceans including the hydrothermal vents, and numerous other ecological niches, including parasitic ones. Although the name "snail" can be, and often is, applied to all the members of this class, commonly this word means only those species with an external shell large enough that the soft parts can withdraw completely into it. Those gastropods without a shell, and those with only a very reduced or internal shell, are usually known as slugs. The marine shelled species of gastropod include edible species such as abalone, conches, periwinkles, whelks, and numerous other sea snails that produce seashells which are coiled in the adult stage, even though in some cases the coiling may not be very visible, for example in cowries. There are also a number of families of species such as all the various limpets, where the shell is coiled only in the larval stage, and is a simple conical structure after that.

Etymology

The word "gastropod" is derived from the Ancient Greek words *ãáóôÞñ (gastér,* stem: *gastr-)* "stomach", and *ðïýò (poús,* stem: *pod-)* "foot", hence stomach-foot. This is an anthropomorphic name, based on the fact that to humans it appears as if snails and slugs crawl on their bellies. In reality, snails and slugs have their stomach, the rest of their digestive system and all the rest of their viscera in a hump on the opposite, dorsal side of the body. In most gastropods this visceral hump is covered by, and contained within, the shell. In the scientific literature, gastropods were described under the vernacular (French) name "gasteropodes" by Georges Cuvier in 1795. The name was later Latinized. The earlier name *univalve* means "one valve" or shell, in contrast to *bivalve* applied to mollusks such as clams and meaning that those animals possess two valves or shells.

Diversity

At all taxonomic levels, gastropods are second only to the insects in terms of their diversity. Gastropods are the class of molluscs which have the greatest numbers of named species. However estimates of the total number of gastropod species vary widely, depending on the cited sources. The number of gastropod species can be ascertained from estimates of the number of described species of Mollusca with accepted names: about 85,000 (minimum 50,000, maximum 120,000). But an estimate of the total number of Mollusca, including undescribed species, is about 240,000 species. The estimate of 85,000 molluscs includes 24,000 described species of terrestrial gastropods.

Different estimates for aquatic gastropods (based on different sources) give about 30,000 species of marine gastropods, and about 5,000 species of freshwater and brackish gastropods. The total number of recently discovered species of freshwater snails is about 4,000. There are 444 recently extinct species of gastropods (extinct since the year 1500), 18 species that are now extinct in the wild (but still existing in captivity) and 69 "possibly extinct" species. The number of prehistoric (fossil) species of gastropods is at least 15,000 species.

Habitat

Some of the more familiar and better-known gastropods are terrestrial gastropods (the land snails and slugs) and some live in freshwater, but more than two thirds of all named species live in a marine environment. Gastropods have a worldwide distribution from the near Arctic and Antarctic zones to the tropics. They have become adapted to almost every kind of existence on earth, having colonized every medium available except the air. In habitats where there is not enough calcium carbonate to build a really solid shell, such as on some acidic soils on land, there are still various species of slugs, and also some snails with a thin translucent shell, mostly or entirely composed of the protein conchiolin.

Snails such as *Sphincterochila boissieri* and *Xerocrassa seetzeni* have adapted to desert conditions, other snails have adapted to an existence in ditches, near deepwater hydrothermal vents, the pounding surf of rocky shores, caves, and many other diverse areas.

Body wall

Some sea slugs are very brightly coloured. This serves either as a warning, when they are poisonous or contain stinging cells, or to camouflage them on the brightly-coloured hydroids, sponges and seaweeds on which many of the species are found. Lateral outgrowths on the body of nudibranchs are called cerata. These contain a part of digestive gland, which is called the diverticula.

Sensory Organs and Nervous System

Sensory organs of gastropods include olfactory organs, eyes, statocysts and mechanoreceptors. Gastropods have no hearing. In terrestrial gastropods (land snails and slugs), the olfactory organs, located on the tips of the 4 tentacles, are the most important sensory organ. The chemosensory organs of opisthobranch marine gastropods are called rhinophores. The majority of gastropods have simple visual organs, eye spots, that are situated either at the tip of the tentacles or the base of the tentacles. However "eyes" in gastropods range from these simple ocelli which cannot process an image being only able to distinguish light and dark, to more complex pit eyes, and even to lens eyes. In land snails and slugs, vision is not the most important sense, because they are mainly nocturnal animals.

The nervous system of gastropods includes the peripheral nervous system and the central nervous system. The central nervous system consist of ganglia connected by nerve cells. It includes paired ganglia: the cerebral ganglia, pedal ganglia, osphradial ganglia, pleural ganglia, parietal ganglia and the visceral ganglia. There are sometimes also buccal ganglia.

Digestive System

The radula of a gastropod is usually adapted to the food that a species eats. The simplest gastropods are the limpets and abalones, herbivores that use their hard radula to rasp at seaweeds on rocks. Many marine gastropods are burrowers, and have a siphon that extends out from the mantle edge. Sometimes the shell has a siphonal canal to accommodate this structure. A siphon enables the animal to draw water into their mantle cavity and over the gill. They use the siphon primarily to "taste" the water to detect prey from a distance. Gastropods with siphons tend to be either predators or scavengers.

Respiratory System

Almost all marine gastropods breathe with a gill, but many freshwater species, and the majority of terrestrial species, have a pallial lung. Gastropods with a lung belong to one group with common descent, the Pulmonata, however, gastropods with gills are paraphyletic.

The respiratory protein in almost all gastropods is hemocyanin, but a pulmonate family Planorbidae have hemoglobin as respiratory protein.

In one large group of sea slugs, the gills are arranged as a rosette of feathery plumes on their backs, which gives rise to their other name, nudibranchs. Some nudibranchs have smooth or warty backs and have no visible gill mechanism, such that respiration may likely take place directly through the skin.

Circulatory System

Gastropods have open circulatory system and the transport fluid is hemolymph. Hemocyanin is present in the hemolymph as the respiratory pigment.

Excretory System

The primary organs of excretion in gastropods are nephridia, which produce either ammonia or uric acid as a waste product. The nephridium also plays an important role in maintaining water balance in freshwater and terrestrial species. Additional organs of excretion, at least in some species, include pericardial glands in the body cavity, and digestive glands opening into the stomach.

Reproductive System

Courtship is a part of mating behaviour in some gastropods including some of the Helicidae. Again, in some land snails, an unusual feature of the reproductive system of gastropods is the presence and utilisation of love darts.

In many marine gastropods other than the opisthobranchs, there are separate sexes; most land gastropods however are hermaphrodites.

Life Cycle

The main aspects of the life cycle of gastropods include:

- Egg laying and the eggs of gastropods
- The Embryonic development of gastropods
- The larvae or larval stadium: some gastropods may be trochophore and/or veliger
- Estivation and hibernation (each of these are present in some gastropods only)
- The growth of gastropods
- Courtship and mating in gastropods: fertilisation is internal or external according to the species. External fertilisation is common in marine gastropods.

Feeding Behaviour

Marine gastropods include some that are herbivores, detritus feeders, predatory carnivores, scavengers, parasites, and also a few ciliary feeders, in which the radula is reduced or absent. Land-dwelling species can chew up leaves, bark, fruit and decomposing animals while marine species can scrape algae off the rocks on the sea floor. In some species that have evolved into endoparasites, such as the eulimid *Thyonicola doglieli*, many of the standard gastropod features are strongly reduced or absent. A few sea slugs are herbivores and some are carnivores. Many have distinct dietary preferences and regularly occur in close association with their food species. Some predatory carnivorous gastropods include, for example: Cone shells, *Testacella*, *Daudebardia*, Ghost slug and others.

Genetics

Gastropods exhibit an important degree of variation in mitochondrial gene organisation when compared to other animals. Main events of gene rearrangement occurred at the origin of Patellogastropoda and Heterobranchia, whereas fewer changes occurred between the ancestors of Vetigastropoda (only tRNAs D, C and N) and Caenogastropoda (a large single inversion, and translocations of the tRNAs D and N). Within Heterobranchia, gene order seems to be relatively conserved and gene rearrangements are mostly related with transposition of tRNA genes.

Geological History

The first gastropods were exclusively marine, with the earliest representatives of the group appearing in the Late Cambrian (*Chippewaella*, *Strepsodiscus*). Early Cambrian forms like *Helcionella* and *Scenella* are no longer considered gastropods, and the tiny coiled *Aldanella* of earliest Cambrian time is probably not even a mollusk. By the Ordovician period the gastropods were a varied group present in a range of aquatic habitats. Commonly, fossil gastropods from the rocks of the early Palaeozoic era are too poorly preserved for accurate identification. Still, the Silurian genus *Poleumita* contains fifteen identified species. Fossil gastropods were less common during the Palaeozoic era than bivalves. Most of the gastropods of the Palaeozoic era belong to primitive groups, a few of which still survive today. By the Carboniferous period many of the shapes seen in living gastropods can be matched in the fossil record, but despite these similarities in appearance the majority of these older forms are not directly related to living forms. It was during the Mesozoic era that the ancestors of many of the living gastropods evolved. One of the earliest known terrestrial (land-dwelling) gastropods is *Maturipupa*, which is found in the Coal Measures of the Carboniferous period in Europe, but relatives of the modern land snails are rare before the Cretaceous period, when the familiar *Helix* first appeared.

In rocks of the Mesozoic era, gastropods are slightly more common as fossils, their shells are often well preserved. Their fossils occur in ancient beds deposited in both freshwater and marine environments. The "Purbeck Marble" of the Jurassic period and the "Sussex Marble" of the early Cretaceous period, which both occur in southern England, are limestones containing the tightly packed remains of the pond snail *Viviparus*. Rocks of the Cenozoic era yield very large numbers of gastropod fossils, many of these fossils being closely related to modern living forms. The diversity of the gastropods increased markedly at the beginning of this era, along with that of the bivalves.

Certain trail-like markings preserved in ancient sedimentary rocks are thought to have been made by gastropods crawling over the soft mud and sand. Although these trails are of debatable origin, some of them do resemble the trails made by living gastropods today. Gastropod fossils may sometimes be confused with ammonites or other shelled cephalopods. An example of this is *Bellerophon* from the limestones of the Carboniferous period in Europe, the shell of which is planispirally coiled and can be mistaken for the shell of a cephalopod. Gastropods are one of the groups that record the changes in fauna caused by the advance and retreat of the Ice Sheets during the Pleistocene epoch.

Taxonomy

Since Darwin, biological taxonomy has attempted to reflect the phylogeny of organisms, i.e. the tree of life. The classifications used in taxonomy attempt to represent the precise interrelatedness of the various taxa. However, the taxonomy of the Gastropoda is constantly being revised and because of this, the versions shown in various texts can differ in major ways. In the older classification of the gastropods, there were four subclasses:

- Opisthobranchia (gills to the right and behind the heart).
- Gymnomorpha (no shell)
- Prosobranchia (gills in front of the heart).
- Pulmonata (with a lung instead of gills)

The taxonomy of the Gastropoda is still under revision, and more and more of the old taxonomy is being abandoned, as the results of DNA studies slowly become clearer. Nevertheless a few of the older terms such as "opisthobranch" and "prosobranch" are still sometimes used in a descriptive way. New insights based on DNA sequencing of gastropods have produced some revolutionary new taxonomic insights. In the case of the Gastropoda, the taxonomy is now gradually being rewritten to embody strictly monophyletic groups (only one lineage of gastropods in each group). Integrating new findings into a working taxonomy will continue to be a challenge in coming years. Consistent ranks within the taxonomy at the level of subclass, superorder, order and suborder have already been abandoned as unworkable.

Ongoing revisions of the higher taxonomic levels are to be expected in the near future. Convergent evolution, which appears to exist at especially high frequency in the Gastropoda class, may account for the observed differences between the older phylogenies which were based on morphological data, and more recent gene-sequencing studies. Main articles: Taxonomy of the Gastropoda (Bouchet & Rocroi, 2005) and Changes in the taxonomy of gastropods since 2005 Bouchet & Rocroi (2005) made sweeping changes in the systematics, resulting in a taxonomy that is a step closer to the evolutionary history of the phylum.

The Bouchet & Rocroi classification system is based partly on the older systems of classification, and partly on new cladistic research. In the past, the taxonomy of gastropods was largely based on phenetic morphological characters of the taxa. The recent advances are more based on molecular characters from DNA and RNA research. This has made the taxonomical ranks and their hierarchy controversial. The debate about these issues is not likely to end soon. In the Bouchet, Rocroi *et al.* taxonomy, the authors have used unranked clades for taxa above the rank of superfamily (replacing the ranks suborder, order, superorder and subclass), while using the traditional Linnaean approach for all taxa below the rank of superfamily. Whenever monophyly has not been tested, or is known to be paraphyletic or polyphyletic, the term "group" or "informal group" has been used. The classification of families into subfamilies is often not well resolved, and should be regarded as the best possible hypothesis. In 2004, Brian Simison and David R. Lindberg showed possible diphyletic origins of the Gastropoda based on mitochondrial gene order and amino acid sequence analyses of complete genes.

Chapter 8

Priapulida: Character and Classification

Priapulida (priapulid worms or penis worms, diminutive) is a phylum of marine worms. They are named for their extensible spiny proboscis, which, in some species, may have a shape like that of a human penis. They live in the mud, which they eat, in comparatively shallow waters up to 90 metres (300 ft). Together with Echiura and Sipuncula, they were once placed in the taxon Gephyrea, but it is now clear that they belong to Ecdysozoa, which mostly include microscopic animals, with the exception of the relatively large arthropods, velvet worms, and the priapulids.

Their nearest relatives are probably Kinorhyncha and Loricifera with which they constitute the taxon Scalidophora. They feed on slow-moving invertebrates, such as polychaete worms. Priapulid-like fossils are known at least as far back as the Middle Cambrian. They were likely major predators of the Cambrian period. However, crown-group priapulids can

Anatomy

Priapulids are cylindrical worm-like animals, ranging from 0.5 to 20 centimetres (0.20 to 7.9 in) in length, with a median anterior mouth quite devoid of any armature or tentacles. The body is divided into a main trunk or abdomen and a somewhat swollen proboscis region ornamented with longitudinal ridges.

The body is ringed and often has circles of spines, which are continued into the slightly protrusible pharynx. Some species may also have a tail or a pair of caudal appendages. The body has a chitinous cuticle that is moulted as the animal grows. There is a wide body-cavity, it has no connection with the renal or reproductive organs, so it is not a coelom; it is probably a blood-space or hemocoel. There are no vascular or respiratory systems, but the body cavity does contain phagocytic amoebocytes and cells containing the respiratory pigment haemerythrin. The alimentary canal is straight, consisting of an eversible pharynx, an intestine, and a short rectum. The pharynx is muscular and lined by teeth. The anus is terminal, although in *Priapulus* one or two hollow ventral diverticula of the body-wall stretch out behind it. The nervous system comprises a nerve ring around the pharynx and a single ventral cord running the length of the body and including a number of ganglia. It retains its primitive connection with the ectoderm, forming part of the body wall. There are no specialised sense organs, but there are sensory nerve endings in the body, especially on the proboscis. The priapulids are gonochoristic, having two separate sexes (i.e. male and female).

Their male and female organs are closely associated with the excretory protonephridia. They comprise a pair of branching tufts, each of which opens to the exterior on one side of the anus. The tips of these tufts enclose a flame-cell like those found in flatworms and other animals, and these probably function as excretory organs. As the animals mature, diverticula arise on the tubes of these organs, which develop either spermatozoa or ova. These sex cells pass out through the ducts.

Fossil Record

Stem-group Priapulids are known from the Middle Cambrian Burgess shale, where their soft-part anatomy is preserved, often in conjunction with their gut contents – allowing a reconstruction of their diets. Trace fossils that are morphologically almost identical to the burrows (*Treptichnus pedum*) officially mark the start of the Cambrian period, suggesting that priapulids, or at least close anatomical relatives, evolved around this time.

Nematode

The nematodes or roundworms (phylum Nematoda) are the most diverse phylum of pseudocoelomates, and one of the most diverse of all animals. Nematode species are very difficult to distinguish; over 28,000 have been described, of which over 16,000 are parasitic. The total number of nematode species has been estimated to be about 1,000,000. Unlike cnidarians or flatworms, roundworms have tubular digestive systems with openings at both ends.

Habitats

Nematodes have successfully adapted to nearly every ecosystem from marine to fresh water, to soils, and from the polar regions to the tropics, as well as the highest to the lowest of elevations. They are ubiquitous in freshwater, marine, and terrestrial environments, where they often outnumber other animals in both individual and species counts, and are found in locations as diverse as mountains, deserts, oceanic trenches, and within the earth's lithosphere.

They represent, for example, 90% of all life forms on the ocean floor. Their numerical dominance, often exceeding more than 1 million individuals per square metre and accounting for about 80% of all individual animals on earth, their diversity in lifestyles and their presence at various trophic levels point at an important role in many ecosystems. Their many parasitic forms include pathogens in most plants and animals (including humans). Some nematodes can undergo cryptobiosis. One group of carnivorous fungi, the nematophagous fungi, are predators of soil nematodes. They set enticements for the nematodes in the form of lassos or adhesive structures.

Nematodes have even been found at great depth (0.9–3.6 km) below the surface of the Earth in gold mines in South Africa. Nathan Cobb (from p. 472 of Cobb, 1914) described the ubiquitous presence of nematodes on Earth as follows:

> *"In short, if all the matter in the universe except the nematodes were swept away, our world would still be dimly recognisable, and if, as disembodied spirits, we could then investigate it, we should find its mountains, hills, vales, rivers, lakes, and oceans represented by a film of nematodes. The location of towns would be decipherable, since for every massing of human beings there would be a corresponding massing*

of certain nematodes. Trees would still stand in ghostly rows representing our streets and highways. The location of the various plants and animals would still be decipherable, and, had we sufficient knowledge, in many cases even their species could be determined by an examination of their erstwhile nematode parasites."

Taxonomy and Systematics

The group was originally defined by Karl Rudolphi in 1808 under the name Nematoidea, from Ancient Greek íÆìá (*nêma, nêmatos*, 'thread') and -eiä ò (*-eidçs*, 'species'). It was reclassified as family Nematodes by Burmeister in 1837 and order Nematoda by K. M. Diesing in 1861. At its origin, the "Nematoidea" included both roundworms and horsehair worms. Along with Acanthocephala, Trematoda and Cestoidea, it formed the group Entozoa. The first differentiation of roundworms from horsehair worms, though erroneous, is due to von Siebold (1843) with orders Nematoidea and Gordiacei (Gordiacea). They were classed along with Acanthocephala in the new phylum Nemathelminthes (today obsolete) by Gegenbaur (1859).

The taxon Nematoidea, including the family Gordiidae (horsehair worms), was then promoted to the rank of phylum by Ray Lankester (1877). In 1919, Nathan Cobb proposed that roundworms should be recognised alone as a phylum. He argued they should be called nema(s) in English rather than "nematodes" and defined the taxon Nemates (Latin plural of *nema*). Since Cobb was the first to exclude all but nematodes from the group, some sources consider the valid taxon name to be Nemates or Nemata, rather than Nematoda.

Phylogeny

The relationships of the nematodes and their close relatives among the protostomian Metazoa are unresolved. Traditionally, they were held to be a lineage of their own, but in the 1990s it was proposed that they form a clade together with moulting animals such as arthropods. This group has been named Ecdysozoa. However, the monophyly of the Ecdysozoa was never unequivocally accepted: while most researchers consider at least the placement of arthropods as close relatives of annelids—with which they were formerly united—to be unwarranted, the presumed close relationships of the nematodes and relatives with the arthropods has been a major point of contention. Even though the amount of data since accumulated in regard to this problem is staggering, the situation seems if anything less clear these days. DNA sequence data, initially strongly supporting the Ecdysozoa hypothesis, have become rather equivocal on ecdysozoan monophyly, and are simply unable to refute either a close or a more distant relationship between the arthropod and nematode lineages.

That the roundworms have a large number of peculiar apomorphies and in many cases a parasitic lifestyle confounds morphological analyses. Genetic analyses of roundworms suggest that—as is also indicated by their unique morphological features—the group has been under intense selective pressure during its early radiation, resulting apparently in accelerated rates of both morphological and molecular evolution. Furthermore, no distinctive apomorphies of Ecdysozoa are known; even moulting has recently been confirmed to occur outside the presumed clade.

Conversely, the identity of the closest living relatives of the Nematoda has always been considered to be well resolved. Morphological characters and molecular phylogenies agree with placement of the roundworms as sister taxon to the parasitic horsehair worms (Nematomorpha); together they make up the Nematoida. Together with the Scalidophora (formerly Cephalorhyncha), the Nematoida form the Introverta. It is entirely unclear whether the Introverta are, in turn, the closest living relatives of the enigmatic Gastrotricha; if so, they are considered a clade Cycloneuralia, but there is much disagreement both between and among the available morphological and molecular data. The Cycloneuralia or the Introverta—depending on the validity of the former—are often ranked as a superphylum.

Nematode Systematics

Due to the lack of knowledge regarding many nematodes, their systematics is contentious. An earliest and influential classification was proposed by Chitwood and Chitwood—later revised by Chitwood—who divided the phylum into two—the

Aphasmidia and the *Phasmidia*. These were later renamed *Adenophorea* (gland bearers) and *Secernentea* (secretors) respectively. The *Secernentea* share several characteristics including the presence of phasmids, a pair of sensory organs located in the lateral posterior region and this was used as the basis for this division. This scheme was adhered to in many later classifications even though it was realised that the *Adenophorea* were not a uniform group. Initial DNA sequence studies suggested the existence of five clades:

- Dorylaimia
- Enoplia
- Spirurina
- Tylenchina
- Rhabditina

As it seems, the Secernentea are indeed a natural group of closest relatives. But the "Adenophorea" appear to be a paraphyletic assemblage of roundworms simply retaining a good number of ancestral traits. The old Enoplia do not seem to be monophyletic either but to contain two distinct lineages. The old group "Chromadoria" seem to be another paraphyletic assemblage, with the Monhysterida representing a very ancient minor group of nematodes. Among the Secernentea, the Diplogasteria may need to be united with the Rhabditia while the Tylenchia might be paraphyletic with the Rhabditia.

The understanding of roundworm systematics and phylogeny as of 2002 is summarised below:

Phylum Nematoda

- Basal order Monhysterida
- Class Dorylaimea
- Class Enoplea
- Class Secernentea
  - Subclass Diplogasteria (disputed)
  - Subclass Rhabditia (paraphyletic?)
  - Subclass Spiruria
  - Subclass Tylenchia (disputed)
- "Chromadorea" assemblage

Later work has suggested the presence of 12 clades. It appears that *Secernentea*—a group that includes virtually all major animal and plant 'nematode' parasites—arose from within the *Adenophorea*. A major effort to improve the systematics of this phylum is in progress and being organised by the 959 Nematode Genomes.

Anatomy

Nematodes are slender worms, typically less than 2.5 millimetres (0.10 in) long. The smallest nematodes are microscopic, while free-living species can reach as much as 5 centimetres (2.0 in) and some parasitic species are larger still, reaching over a metre in length. The body is often ornamented with ridges, rings, bristles or other distinctive structures.

The head of a nematode is relatively distinct. Whereas the rest of the body is bilaterally symmetrical, the head is radially symmetrical, with sensory bristles and, in many cases, solid 'head-shields' radiating outwards around the mouth. The mouth has either three or six lips, which often bear a series of teeth on their inner edges.

An adhesive 'caudal gland' is often found at the tip of the tail. The epidermis is either a syncytium or a single layer of cells, and is covered by a thick collagenous cuticle. The cuticle is often of complex structure, and may have two or three distinct layers. Underneath the epidermis lies a layer of muscle cells. Projections run from the inner surface of these cells towards the nerve cords; this is a unique arrangement in the animal kingdom, in which nerve cells normally extend fibres into the muscles rather than *vice versa*.

Nervous System

Four peripheral nerves run the length of the body on the dorsal, ventral, and lateral surfaces. Each nerve lies within a cord of connective tissue lying beneath the cuticle and between the muscle cells. The ventral nerve is the largest, and has a double structure forward of the excretory pore. The dorsal nerve is responsible for motor control, while the lateral nerves are sensory, and the ventral combines both functions. At the anterior end of the animal, the nerves branch from a dense, circular nerve ring surrounding the pharynx, and serving as the brain. Smaller nerves run forward from the ring to supply the sensory organs of the head. The body of nematodes is covered in numerous sensory bristles and papillae that together provide a sense of touch. Behind the sensory bristles on the head lie two small pits, or 'amphids'. These are well supplied with nerve cells, and are probably chemoreception organs. A few aquatic nematodes possess what appear to be pigmented eye-spots, but is unclear whether or not these are actually sensory in nature.

Reproduction

Most nematode species are dioecious, with separate male and female individuals. Both sexes possess one or two tubular gonads. In males, the sperm are produced at the end of the gonad, and migrate along its length as they mature. The testes each open into a relatively wide sperm duct and then into a glandular and muscular ejaculatory duct associated with the cloaca. In females, the ovaries each open into an oviduct and then a glandular uterus.

The uteri both open into a common vagina, usually located in the middle of the ventral surface. Reproduction is usually sexual. Males are usually smaller than females (often much smaller) and often have a characteristically bent tail for holding the female for copulation. During copulation, one or more chitinized spicules move out of the cloaca and are inserted into genital pore of the female. Amoeboid sperm crawl along the spicule into the female worm. Nematode sperm is thought to be the only eukaryotic cell without the globular protein G-actin.

Eggs may be embryonated or unembryonated when passed by the female, meaning their fertilized eggs may not yet be developed. A few species are known to be ovoviviparous. The eggs are protected by an outer shell, secreted by the uterus. In free-living roundworms, the eggs hatch into larvae, which appear essentially identical to the adults, except for an underdeveloped reproductive system; in parasitic roundworms, the life cycle is often much more complicated.

Nematodes as a whole possess a wide range of modes of reproduction. Some nematodes, such as *Heterorhabditis* spp., undergo a process called *endotokia matricida*: intrauterine birth causing maternal death. Some nematodes are hermaphroditic, and keep their self-fertilized eggs inside the uterus until they hatch. The juvenile nematodes will then ingest the parent nematode. This process is significantly promoted in environments with a low or reducing food supply.

The nematode model species *Caenorhabditis elegans* and *C. briggsae* exhibit and rodioecy, which is very rare among animals. The single genus *Meloidogyne* (root-knot nematodes) exhibit a range of reproductive modes, including sexual reproduction, facultative sexuality (in which most, but not all, generations reproduce asexually), and both meiotic and mitotic parthenogenesis. The genus *Mesorhabditis* exhibits an unusual form of parthenogenesis, in which sperm-producing males copulate with females, but the sperm do not fuse with the ovum. Contact with the sperm is essential for the ovum to begin dividing, but because there is no fusion of the cells, the male contributes no genetic material to the offspring, which are essentially clones of the female.

Free-Living Species

In free-living species, development usually consists of four molts of the cuticle during growth. Different species feed on materials as varied as algae, fungi, small animals, fecal matter, dead organisms and living tissues. Free-living marine nematodes are important and abundant members of the meiobenthos. They play an important role in the decomposition process, aid in recycling of nutrients in marine environments and are sensitive to changes in the environment caused by pollution. One roundworm of note, *Caenorhabditis elegans*, lives in the soil and has found much use as a model organism. *C. elegans* has had its entire genome sequenced, as well as the developmental fate of every cell determined, and every neuron mapped.

Parasitic Species

Nematodes commonly parasitic on humans include ascarids (*Ascaris*), filarias, hookworms, pinworms (*Enterobius*) and whipworms (*Trichuris trichiura*). The species *Trichinella spiralis*, commonly known as the 'trichina worm', occurs in rats, pigs, and humans, and is responsible for the disease trichinosis. *Baylisascaris* usually infests wild animals, but can be deadly to humans, as well. *Dirofilaria immitis* heartworms are known for causing heartworm disease by inhabiting the hearts, arteries, and lungs of dogs and some cats. *Haemonchus contortus* is one of the most abundant infectious agents in sheep around the world, causing great economic damage to sheep farms. In contrast, entomopathogenic nematodes parasitize insects and are considered by humans to be beneficial.

One form of nematode is entirely dependent upon fig wasps, which are the sole source of fig fertilization. They prey upon the wasps, riding them from the ripe fig of the wasp's birth to the fig flower of its death, where they kill the wasp, and their offspring await the birth of the next generation of wasps as the fig ripens.

A newly discovered parasitic tetradonematid nematode, *Myrmeconema neotropicum*, apparently induces fruit mimicry in the tropical ant *Cephalotes atratus*. Infected ants develop bright red gasters, tend to be more sluggish, and walk with their gasters in a conspicuous elevated position. These changes likely cause frugivorous birds to confuse the infected ants for berries, and eat them. Parasite eggs passed in the bird's feces are subsequently collected by foraging *Cephalotes atratus* and are fed to their larvae, thus completing the life cycle of *M. neotropicum*.

Plant-parasitic nematodes include several groups causing severe crop losses. The most common genera are *Aphelenchoides* (foliar nematodes), *Ditylenchus*, *Globodera* (potato cyst nematodes), *Heterodera* (soybean cyst nematodes), *Longidorus*, *Meloidogyne* (root-knot nematodes), *Nacobbus*, *Pratylenchus* (lesion nematodes), *Trichodorus* and *Xiphinema* (dagger nematodes).

Several phytoparasitic nematode species cause histological damages to roots, including the formation of visible galls (e.g. by root-knot nematodes), which are useful characters for their diagnostic in the field. Some nematode species transmit plant viruses through their feeding activity on roots. One of them is *Xiphinema index*, vector of grapevine fanleaf virus), an important disease of grapes.

Other nematodes attack bark and forest trees. The most important representative of this group is *Bursaphelenchus xylophilus*, the pine wood nematode, present in Asia and America and recently discovered in Europe.

Agriculture and Horticulture

Depending on the species, a nematode may be beneficial or detrimental to plant health. From agricultural and horticulture perspectives, the two categories of nematode: predatory ones, which will kill garden pests like cutworms, and pest nematodes, like the root-knot nematode, which attack plants and those that act as vectors spreading plant viruses between crop plants. Predatory nematodes can be bred by soaking a specific recipe of leaves and other detritus in water, in a dark, cool place, and can even be purchased as an organic form of pest control. Rotations of plants with nematode resistant species or varieties is one means of managing parasitic nematode infestations. For example, marigolds, grown over one or more seasons (the effect is cumulative), can be used to control nematodes. Another is treatment with natural antagonists such as the fungus *Gliocladium roseum*. Chitosan is a natural biocontrol that elicits plant defence responses to destroy parasitic cyst nematodes on roots of soybean, corn, sugar beet, potato and tomato crops without harming beneficial nematodes in the soil. Furthermore, soil steaming is an efficient method to kill nematodes before planting the crop, but indiscriminately eliminates both harmful and beneficial ones. CSIRO has found a 13- to 14-fold reduction of nematode population densities in plots having Indian mustard (*Brassica juncea*) green manure or seed meal in the soil. Hundreds of *Caenorhabditis elegans* were featured in a research project on NASA's STS-107 space mission, and were the only known living organisms to have survived the Space Shuttle Columbia Disaster.

Nematomorpha

Nematomorpha (sometimes called Gordiacea, and commonly known as horsehair worms or Gordian worms) is a phylum of parasitic animals that are superficially morphologically similar to nematode worms, hence the name. They range in size in most species from 50 to 100 centimetres (20 to 39 in) long and can reach in extreme cases up to 2 metres, and 1 to 3 millimetres (0.039 to 0.12 in) in diametre. Horsehair worms can be discovered in damp areas such as watering troughs, streams, puddles, and cisterns. The adult worms are free living, but the larvae are parasitic on beetles, cockroaches, orthopterans, and crustaceans. About 351 species are known and a conservative estimate suggests that there may be about 2000 species worldwide. The name "Gordian" stems from the legendary Gordian knot. This relates to the fact that nematomorpha often tie themselves in knots.

Description and Biology

Nematomorphs possess an external cuticle without cilia. Internally, they have only longitudinal muscle and a non-functional gut, with no excretory, respiratory or circulatory systems. The nervous system consists of a nerve ring near the anterior end of the animal, and a ventral nerve cord running along the body. Reproductively, they are dioecious, with the internal fertilization of eggs that are then laid in gelatinous strings. Adults have cylindrical gonads, opening into the cloaca. The larvae have rings of cuticular hooks and terminal stylets that are believed to be used to enter the hosts. Once inside the host, the larvae live inside the haemocoel and absorb nutrients directly through their skin. Development into the adult form takes weeks or months, and the larva moults several times as it grows in size. The adults are mostly free living in freshwater or marine environments, and males and females aggregate into tight balls (*Gordian knots*) during mating. In *Spinochordodes tellinii*, which has orthopterans as its vector, the infection acts on the insect's brain and causes it to seek water and drown itself, thus returning the nematomorph to water. They are also remarkably able to survive the predation of their host, being able to wriggle out of the predator that has eaten the host.

Taxonomy

Nematomorphs can be confused with nematodes, particularly mermithid worms. Unlike nematomorphs, mermithids do not have a terminal cloaca. Male mermithids have one or two spicules just before the end apart from having a thinner, smoother cuticle, without areoles and a paler brown colour. The phylum is placed along with the Ecdysozoa clade of moulting organisms that include the Arthropoda. Fossilized worms have been reported from Early Cretaceous. Burmese amber dated to 100–110 million years. Relationships within the phylum are still somewhat unclear, but two classes are recognised. The five marine species of nematomorph are contained in Nectonematoida. Adults are planktonic and the larvae parasitise decapod crustaceans, especially crabs. They are characterised by a double row of natotory setae along each side of the body, dorsal and ventral longitudinal epidermal cords, a spacious and fluid-filled blastocoelom and singular gonads. The approximately 320 remaining species are distributed into two families and seven genera within order Gordioida. Gordioidean adults are free-living in freshwater or semiterrestrial habitats and larvae parasitise insects, primarily orthopterans. Unlike nectonematiodeans, gordioideans lack lateral rows of setae, have a single, ventral epidermal cord and their blastocoels are filled with mesenchyme in young animals but become spacious in older individuals.

Entoprocta

Entoprocta, whose name means "anus inside", is a phylum of mostly sessile aquatic animals, ranging from 0.1 to 7 millimetres (0.0039 to 0.28 in) long. Mature individuals are goblet-shaped, on relatively long stalks. They have a "crown" of solid tentacles whose cilia generate water currents that draw food particles towards the mouth, and both the mouth and anus lie inside the "crown". The superficially similar Bryozoa (Ectoprocta) have the anus outside a "crown" of hollow tentacles. Most families of entoprocts are colonial, and all but 2 of the 150 species are marine. A few solitary species can move slowly.

Some species eject unfertilized ova into the water, while others keep their ova in brood chambers until they hatch, and some of these species use placenta-like organs to nourish the developing eggs. After hatching, the larvae swim for a short time and then settle on a surface.

There they metamorphose, and the larval gut generally rotates by up to 180°, so that the mouth and anus face upwards. Both colonial and solitary species also reproduce by cloning – solitary species grow clones in the space between the tentacles and then release them when developed, while colonial ones produce new members from the stalks or from corridor-like stolons. Nudibranchs ("sea slugs") of the genus Trapania and turbellarian flatworms prey on entoprocts. A few entoproct species have been found living in close association with other animals. It is uncertain whether any are invasive species.

Fossils of entoprocts are very rare, and the earliest specimens that have been identified with confidence date from the Late Jurassic. Most studies from 1996 onwards have regarded entoprocts as members of the Trochozoa, which also includes molluscs and annelids. However, a study in 2008 concluded that entoprocts are closely related to bryozoans.

Names

"Entoprocta", coined in 1870, means "anus inside". The alternative name "Kamptozoa", meaning "bent" or "curved" animals, was assigned in 1929. Some authors use "Entoprocta", while others prefer "Kamptozoa".

Description

Most species are colonial, and their members are known as "zooids", since they are not fully independent animals. Zooids are typically 1 millimetre (0.039 in) long but ranging from 0.1 to 7 millimetres (0.0039 to 0.28 in) long.

Zooids

The body of a mature entoproct zooid has a goblet-like structure with a calyx mounted on a relatively long stalk that attaches to a surface. The rim of the calyx bears a "crown" of 8 to 30 solid tentacles, which are extensions of the body wall. The base of the "crown" of tentacles is surrounded by a membrane that partially covers the tentacles when they retract. The mouth and anus lie on opposite sides of the atrium (space enclosed by the "crown" of tentacles), and both can be closed by sphincter muscles. The gut is U-shaped, curving down towards the base of the calyx, where it broadens to form the stomach. This is lined with a membrane consisting of a single layer of cells, each of which has multiple cilia. The stalks of colonial species arise from shared attachment plates or from a network of stolons, tubes that run across a surface. In solitary species the stalk ends in a muscular sucker, or a flexible foot, or is cemented to a surface. The stalk is muscular and produces a characteristic nodding motion. In some species it is segmented. Some solitary species can move, either by creeping on the muscular foot or by somersaulting.

The body wall consists of the epidermis and an external cuticle, which consists mainly of criss-cross collagen fibres. The epidermis contains only a single layer of cells, each of which bears multiple cilia ("hairs") and microvilli (tiny "pleats") that penetrate through the cuticle. The stolons and stalks of colonial species have thicker cuticles, stiffened with chitin. There is no coelom (internal fluid-filled cavity lined with peritoneum) and the other internal organs are embedded in connective tissue that lies between the stomach and the base of the "crown" of tentacles. The nervous system runs through the connective tissue and just below the epidermis, and is controlled by a pair of ganglia. Nerves run from these to the calyx, tentacles and stalk, and to sense organs in all these areas.

Feeding, Digestion, Excretion, Circulation and Respiration

A band of cells, each with multiple cilia, runs along the sides of the tentacles, connecting each tentacle to its neighbours, except that there is a gap in the band nearest the anus. A separate band of cilia runs along a groove that runs close to the inner side of the base of the "crown", with a narrow extension up the inner surface of each tentacle. The cilia on the sides of the tentacles create a current that flows into the "crown" at the bases of the tentacles and exits above the centre of the "crown". These cilia pass food particles to the cilia on the inner surface of the tentacles, and the inner cillia produce a downward current that drives particles into and round the groove, and then to the mouth. Entoprocts generally use one or both of: ciliary sieving, in which one band of cilia creates the feeding current and another traps food particles (the "seive"); and downstream collecting, in which food articles are trapped as they are about to exit past them. In entoprocts, downstream collecting is done by the same bands of cilia that generate the current; trochozoan larvae also use downstream collecting, but use a separate set of cilia to trap food particles.

In addition glands in the tentacles secrete sticky threads that capture large particles. A non-colonial species reported from around the Antarctic Peninsula in 1993 has cells that superficially resemble the cnidocytes of cnidaria, and fire sticky threads. These unusual cells lie around the mouth, and may provide an additional means of capturing prey.

The stomach and intestine are lined with microvilli, which are thought to absorb nutrients. The anus, which opens inside the “crown”, ejects solid wastes into the outgoing current after the tentacles have filtered food out of the water; in some families it is raised on a cone above the level of the groove that conducts food to the mouth.

Most species have a pair of protonephridia which extract soluble wastes from the internal fluids and eliminate them through pores near the mouth. However the freshwater species *Urnatella gracilis* has multiple nephridia in the calyx and stalk. The zooids absorb oxygen and emit carbon dioxide by diffusion, which works well for small animals.

Evolutionary History

Fossil Record

Since entoprocts are small and soft-bodied, fossils have been extremely rare. In 1977 Simon Conway Morris provided the first description of *Dinomischus*, a sessile animal with calyx, stalk and holdfast, found in Canada’s Burgess Shale, which was formed about 505 million years ago. Morris regarded this animal as the earliest known entoproct, since its mouth and anus lay inside a ring of structures above the calyx, but noted that these structures were flat and rather stiff, while the tentacles of modern entoprocts are flexible and have a round cross-section. In 1992 J.A. Todd and P.D. Taylor concluded that *Dinomischus* was not an entoproct, because it did not have the typical rounded, flexible tentacles and the fossils showed no other features that clearly resembled those of entoprocts. In their opinion the earliest fossil entoprocts were specimens they found from Late Jurassic rocks in England. These resemble the modern colonial genus *Barentsia* in many ways, including: upright zooids linked by a network of stolons encrusting the surface to which the colony is attached; straight stalks joined to the stolons by bulky sockets with transverse bands of wrinkles; overall size and proportions similar to that of modern species of *Barentsia*.

Family Tree

When entoprocts were discovered in the nineteenth century, they and bryozoans (ectoprocts) were regarded as classes within the phylum Bryozoa, because both groups were sessile animals that filter-fed by means of a “crown” of tentacles that bore cilia.

However, from 1869 onwards increasing awareness of differences, including the position of the entoproct anus inside the feeding structure and the difference in the early pattern of division of cells in their embryos, caused scientists to regard the two groups as separate phyla.

"Bryozoa" then became just an alternative name for ectoprocts, in which the anus is outside the feeding organ. However studies by one team in 2007 and 2008 argues for sinking Entoprocta into Bryozoa as a class, and resurrecting *Ectoprocta* as a name for the currently identified bryozoans. The consensus of studies from 1996 onwards has been that entoprocts are part of the Trochozoa, a protostome "superphylum" whose members are united in having as their most basic larval form the trochophore type. The trochozoa also include molluscs, annelids, flatworms, nemertines and others. However, scientists disagree about which phylum is mostly closely related to enctoprocts within the trochozoans. An analysis in 2008 re-introduced the pre-1869 meaning of the term "Bryozoa", for a group in which entoprocts and ectoprocts are each other's closest relatives.

Gymnolaemata

Gymnolaemata is a class of the phylum Bryozoa. Gymnolaemata typically live under seawater and grow on surfaces of rocks, kelps, and even in some cases, on animal species like fish. They are mostly marine bryozoans with cylindrical or flattened zooids. The lophophore is protruded by action of muscles pulling on frontal wall. This order includes the majority of living bryozoan species.

Phoronid

Phoronids (scientific name Phoronida) are a phylum of marine animals that filter-feed with a lophophore (a "crown" of tentacles), and build upright tubes of chitin to support and protect their soft bodies. They live in all the oceans and seas including the Arctic Ocean but excluding the Antarctic Ocean, and between the intertidal zone and about 400 metres down. Most adult phoronids are 2 cm long and about 1.5 mm wide, although the largest are 50 cm long. The bottom end of the body is an ampulla (a flask-like swelling), which anchors the animal in the tube and enables it to retract its body very quickly when threatened. When the lophophore is extended at the top of the body, cilia (little hairs) on the sides of the tentacles draw food particles to the mouth, which is inside and slightly to one side of the base of the lophophore.

Unwanted material can be excluded by closing a lid above the mouth or be rejected by the tentacles, whose cilia can switch into reverse. The food then moves down to the stomach, which is in the ampulla. Solid wastes are moved up the intestine and out through the anus, which is outside and slightly below the lophophore. A blood vessel leads up the middle of the body from the stomach to a circular vessel at the base of the lophophore, and from there a single blind vessel runs up each tentacle. A pair of blood vessels near the body wall lead downward from the lophophore ring to the stomach and also to blind branches throughout the body. There is no heart, but the major vessels can contract in waves to move the blood. Phoronids do not ventilate their trunks with oxygenated water, but rely on respiration through the lophophore. The blood contains hemoglobin, which is unusual in such small animals and seems to be an adaptation to anoxic and hypoxic environments. The blood of *Phoronis architecta* carries twice as much oxygen as a human of the same weight. Two metanephridia filter the body fluid, returning any useful products and dumping the remaining soluble wastes through a pair of pores beside the anus.

One species builds colonies by budding or by splitting into top and bottom sections, and all phoronids reproduce sexually from spring to autumn. The eggs of most species form free-swimming actinotroch larvae, which feed on plankton. An actinotroch settles to the seabed after about 20 days and then undergoes a radical change in 30 minutes: the larval tentacles are replaced by the adult lophophore; the anus moves from the bottom to just outside the lophophore; and this changes the gut from upright to a U-bend, with the stomach at the bottom of the body. One species forms a "slug-like" larva, and the larvae of a few species are not known. Phoronids live for about one year. Some species live separately, in vertical tubes embedded in soft sediment, while others form tangled masses buried in or encrusting rocks and shells. In some habitats populations of phoronids reach tens of thousand of individuals per square metre. The actinotroch larvae are familiar among plankton, and sometimes account for a significant proportion of the zooplankton biomass. Predators include fish, gastropods (snails), and nematodes (tiny roundworms). One phoronid species is unpalatable to many epibenthic predators. Various parasites infest phoronids' body cavities, digestive tract and tentacles. It is unknown whether phoronids have any significance for humans. The International Union for Conservation of Nature (IUCN) has not listed any phoronid species as endangered. As of 2010 there are no indisputable body fossils of phoronids. There is good evidence that phoronids created trace fossils found in the Silurian, Devonian, Permian, Jurassic and Cretaceous periods, and possibly in the Ordovician and Triassic. Phoronids, brachiopods and bryozoans (ectoprocts) have collectively been called lophophorates, because all use lophophores to feed. From about the 1940s to the 1990s, family trees based on embryological and morphological features placed lophophorates among or as a sister group to the deuterostomes, a super-phylum which includes chordates and echinoderms. While a minority adhere to this view, most researchers now regard phoronids as members of the protosome super-phylum Lophotrochozoa. Although analysts using molecular phylogeny are confident that members of Lophotrochozoa are more closely related to each other than of non-members, the relationships between members are mostly unclear. Some analyses regard phoronids and brachiopods as sister-groups, while others place phoronids as a sub-group within brachiopoda.

Bibliography

Alexander, R. McN.: *Camparative Vertebrates*, Cambridge University Press, London, 1995.

Anderson, D. T.: *Invertebrate zoology,* Oxford University Press, Oxford, 2019.

Beckner, M.: *The Biological Way of Thought*, University of California Press, Berkeley and Los Angeles, 2008.

Brusca, R. C., & Brusca, G. J.: *Invertebrates,* Sinauer Associates, Sunderland, Mass, 2018.

Campbell, Neil A.; Brad Williamson; Robin J. Heyden: *Biology: Exploring Life*, Pearson Prentice Hall, Boston, Massachusetts, 2016.

Dams, R.D.: *Principles of Neurology*, McGraw Hill, New York, 2007.

Fritz, A.: *International Classification of Diseases for Oncology*, World Health Organization, Geneva, 2023.

Gaskell, W. H.: *The Origin of Vertebrates*, Longman, London, 1998.

Haubrich, W.S.: *Bockus Gastroenterology*, Saunders, Philadelphia, 2015.

Jameson, J. L.: *Principles of Molecular Medicine*, Humana Press, Totowa, 2018.

Kallenbach, N.R.: *Molecular Structure: Chemical Reactivity and Biological Activity,* Oxford University Press, Oxford, 2008.

Lambers, H.: *Plant Physiological Ecology*, Springer-Verlag, New York, 2018.

Manning, M. J.: *Phylogeny of Immunological Memory, Developments in Immunology*. Amsterdam, Biomedical Press, Elsevier/North-Holland, 2000.

Neff, H.: *Chemical Characterization of Ceramic Pastes in Archaeology*, Prehistory Press, Madison, WI, 2012.

Ohno, S.: *Primordial Immunity: Foundations for the Vertebrate Immune System*, New York, New York Academy of Sciences, 2014.

Panchen, A. L.: *The Terrestrial Environment and the Origin of Land Vertebrates*, Academic Press, New York, 2010.

Richards, O. W.; Davies, R.G.: *Imms' General Textbook of Entomology: Volume 1: Structure, Physiology and Development, Classification and Biology*, Springer, Berlin, 1997.

Schmid-Hempel, Paul: *Parasites in social insects*, Princeton University Press, 2018.

Tarlo, L. B. H.: *Calcified tissues in the earliest vertebrates*, Cambridge University Press, London, 2005.

Vetvicka, V., Síma, P., Cooper, E. L., Bilej, M. and Roch, P.: *Immunology of Annelids*. CRC Press, Boca Raton, 2014.

Wallace, Robert A., Jack L. King, and Gerald P. Sanders: *Biology: The Science of Life*, Scott, Foreman and Company, Glenview, IL, 2006.

Walls, G. L.: 1992, The Vertebrate Eye and its Adaptive Radiation: Bloomfield Hills, Michigan, The Cranbrook Institute of Science.

Warr, G. W. and Cohen, N.: *Phylogenesis of Immune Functions*. CRC Press, Boca Raton, 2011.

Index

H

I

J

L

M

N

P

R

S

T

V